Begin Hairdressing & Barbering

Revised 2nd Edition

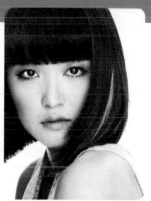

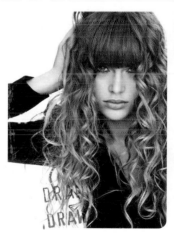

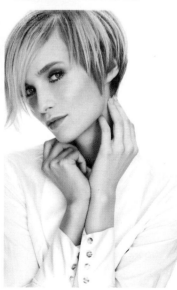

SCOTT SMURTHWAITE @ CREAM

HABIA SERIES LIST

Hairdressing

Student textbooks

Begin Hairdressing: The Official Guide to Level 1 2e *Martin Green*

Hairdressing – The Foundations: The Official Guide to Level 2 6e *Leo Palladino and Martin Green*

Professional Hairdressing: The Official Guide to Level 3 6e *Martin Green and Leo Palladino*

The Official Guide to the City & Guilds Certificate in Salon Services 1e *John Armstrong with Anita Crosland, Martin Green and Lorraine Nordmann*

The Colour Book: The Official Guide to Colour for NVQ Levels 2 and 3 1e *Tracey Lloyd with Christine McMillan-Bodell*

eXtensions: The Official Guide to Hair Extensions 1e *Theresa Bullock*

Salon Management *Martin Green*

Men's Hairdressing: Traditional and Modern Barbering 2e *Maurice Lister*

African-Caribbean Hairdressing 2e *Sandra Gittens*

The World of Hair Colour 1e *John Gray*

The Cutting Book: The Official Guide to Cutting at S/NVQ Levels 2 and 3 *Jane Goldsbro and Elaine White*

Professional Hairdressing titles

Trevor Sorbie: The Bridal Hair Book 1e *Trevor Sorbie and Jacki Wadeson*

The Art of Dressing Long Hair 1e *Guy Kremer and Jacki Wadeson*

Patrick Cameron: Dressing Long Hair 1e *Patrick Cameron and Jacki Wadeson*

Patrick Cameron: Dressing Long Hair 2 1e *Patrick Cameron and Jacki Wadeson*

Bridal Hair 1e *Pat Dixon and Jacki Wadeson*

Professional Men's Hairdressing: The art of cutting and styling 1e *Guy Kremer and Jacki Wadeson*

Essensuals, The Next Generation Toni and Guy: Step by Step 1e *Sacha Mascolo, Christian Mascolo and Stuart Wesson*

Mahogany Hairdressing: Steps to Cutting, Colouring and Finishing Hair 1e *Martin Gannon and Richard Thompson*

Mahogany Hairdressing: Advanced Looks 1e *Martin Gannon and Richard Thompson*

The Total Look: The Style Guide for Hair and Make-Up Professionals 1e *Ian Mistlin*

Trevor Sorbie: Visions in Hair 1e *Trevor Sorbie, Kris Sorbie and Jacki Wadeson*

The Art of Hair Colouring 1e *David Adams and Jacki Wadeson*

Beauty therapy

Beauty Basics: The Official Guide to Level 1 1e *Lorraine Nordmann*

Beauty Therapy – The Foundations: The Official Guide to Level 2 3e *Lorraine Nordmann*

Professional Beauty Therapy – The Official Guide to Level 3 2e *Lorraine Nordmann*

The Official Guide to the City & Guilds Certificate in Salon Services 1e *John Armstrong with Anita Crosland, Martin Green and Lorraine Nordmann*

The Complete Guide to Make-Up 1e *Suzanne Le Quesne*

The Complete Make-Up Artist 2e *Penny Delamar*

The Encyclopedia of Nails 1e *Jacqui Jefford and Anne Swain*

The Art of Nails: A Comprehensive Style Guide to Nail Treatments and Nail Art 1e *Jacqui Jefford*

Nail Artistry 1e *Jacqui Jefford*

The Complete Nail Technician 2e *Marian Newman*

Manicure, Pedicure and Advanced Nail Techniques 1e *Elaine Almond*

The Official Guide to Body Massage 2e *Adele O'Keefe*

An Holistic Guide to Massage 1e *Tina Parsons*

Indian Head Massage 2e *Muriel Burnham-Airey and Adele O'Keefe*

Aromatherapy for the Beauty Therapist 1e *Valerie Worwood*

An Holistic Guide to Reflexology 1e *Tina Parsons*

An Holistic Guide to Anatomy and Physiology 1e *Tina Parsons*

The Essential Guide to Holistic and Complementary Therapy 1e *Helen Beckmann and Suzanne Le Quesne*

The Spa Book 1e *Jane Crebbin-Bailey, Dr John Harcup and John Harrington*

SPA: The Official Guide to Spa Therapy at Levels 2 and 3 *Joan Scott and Andrea Harrison*

Nutrition: A Practical Approach 1e *Suzanne Le Quesne*

Hands on Sports Therapy 1e *Keith Ward*

Encyclopedia of Hair Removal: A Complete Reference to Methods, Techniques and Career Opportunities *Gill Morris and Janice Brown*

The Anatomy and Physiology Workbook: For Beauty and Holistic Therapies Levels 1-3 *Tina Parsons*

The Anatomy and Physiology CD-Rom

Beautiful Selling: The Complete Guide to Sales Success in the Salon *Ruth Langley*

THE **OFFICIAL** GUIDE TO LEVEL 1, REVISED 2E

Begin Hairdressing
& Barbering

Revised 2nd Edition

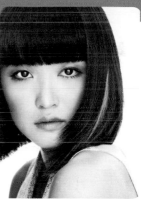

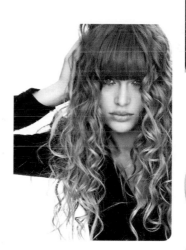

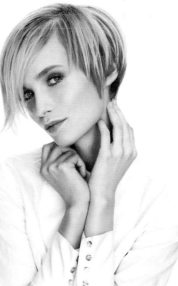

Martin Green

SCOTT SMURTHWAITE @ CREAM

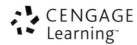
CENGAGE
Learning™

Australia • Brazil • Japan • Korea • Mexico • Singapore • Spain • United Kingdom • United States

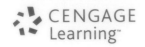

Begin Hairdressing & Barbering – The official guide to Level 1, Revised 2e
Martin Green

Publisher: Melody Dawes

Development Editor: Lucy Mills

Content Project Editor: Lucy Arthy

Editorial assistant: Claire Napoli

Production Controller: Tom Relf

Marketing Executive: Lauren Redwood

Typesetter: MPS Limited, a Macmillan Company

Cover design: HCT Creative

Text design: Design Deluxe

© 2011, Milady, a part of Cengage Learning.

For product information and technology assistance, contact **emea.info@cengage.com**

For permission to use material from this text or product, and for permission queries, email **clsuk.permissions@cengage.com.**

DISCLAIMER

This publication has been developed by Cengage Learning. It is intended as a method of studying for the Habia qualifications. Cengage Learning has taken all reasonable care in the preparation of this publication but Cengage Learning and the City & Guilds of London Institute accept no liability howsoever in respect of any breach of the rights of any third party howsoever occasioned or damage caused to any third party as a result of the use of this publication.

This work is adapted from Begin Hairdressing, 1st Edition, published by Delmar, a division of Cengage Learning, Inc. ©2005.

Cover image kindly supplied by Lee Moran @ Sanrizz, L'Uomo Sculpture Collection

British Library Cataloguing-in-Publication Data
A catalogue record for this book is available from the British Library.

ISBN: 978-1-4080-3979-3

Cengage Learning EMEA
Cheriton House, North Way, Andover
Hampshire. SP10 5BE, UK

Cengage Learning products are represented in Canada by Nelson Education Ltd.

For your lifelong learning solutions, visit **www.cengage.co.uk**

Purchase your next print book, e-book or e-chapter at **www.cengagebrain.com**

Printed by RR Donnelley, China
1 2 3 4 5 6 7 8 9 10 – 12 11 10

Contents

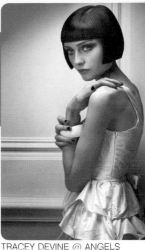

TRACEY DEVINE @ ANGELS

ix Foreword
x Acknowledgements
xii Introduction
xiii Qualification information
xvii About the book
xx FKU mapping grids

Part**one**

2 **The workplace**

Chapter**one**

4 **G20 Make sure your own actions reduce risks to health and safety**

4 Unit G20: quick overview
4 What do I need to do for G20.1?
4 What do I need to do for G20.2?
4 What things do I need to know and understand?
5 Introduction
6 **G20.1 Identify the hazards and evaluate the risks in your workplace**

7 Thinking about your work routines
7 Being responsible
8 Your concerns or questions
9 **G20.2 Reduce the risks to health and safety**

9 Carrying out your duties safely
11 Working in a safe way at all times
16 Risks to health and safety
19 Dressing and behaving professionally
22 Working in an environmentally friendly way
22 Checkerboard
22 Revision questions

Chapter**two**

23 **G3 Contribute to the development of effective working relationships**

23 Unit G3: quick overview

23 What do I need to do for G3.1?
23 What do I need to do for G3.2?
23 What do I need to do for G3.3?
24 What things do I need to cover?
24 What things do I need to know?
24 Introduction
25 **G3.1 Develop effective working relationships with clients**

25 Do things in a way that gives people confidence in your abilities
26 Put clients' belongings away carefully
27 Provide help to others without having to wait to be asked
27 Help clients if they need anything
27 Dress and behave professionally
29 **G3.2 Develop effective working relationships with colleagues**

29 Be friendly, helpful and respectful
29 Ask politely when you need help
30 Help willingly and promptly when asked
30 Only do jobs that you have been trained to do
31 Tell your supervisor about any problems
31 **G3.3 Develop yourself within the job role**

31 Being able to gauge your own abilities
31 Asking other staff when you aren't sure
32 Learning new things
32 Reviewing your progress
35 Checkerboard
35 Revision questions

Chapter**three**

36 **G2 Assist with salon reception duties**

36 Unit G2: quick overview
36 What do I need to do for G2.1?
36 What do I need to do for G2.2?
36 What do I need to do for G2.3?
37 What things do I need to cover?
37 What things do I need to know?
37 Introduction

38 **G2.1** Maintain the reception area

38 Keeping all areas clean and tidy

39 Monitoring stationery and product levels

40 Looking out for faulty or damaged products

40 Demonstrating good customer care

41 **G2.2** Attend to clients and enquiries

41 Handling enquiries politely and positively

42 Informing the stylists that their clients have arrived

43 Referring enquiries you can't handle

43 Taking messages for others

44 Handling information in a confidential way

45 **G2.3** Help to make appointments for salon services

46 Dealing with requests promptly and politely

46 Accurately recording appointments

48 Requesting assistance when needed

48 Confirming and recording details correctly

49 Checkerboard

49 Revision questions

Part**two**

50 **Hairdressing practical skills**

Chapter**four**

52 **GH3 Prepare for hair services and maintain work areas**

52 Unit GH3: quick overview

52 What do I need to do for GH3.1?

52 What do I need to do for GH3.2?

52 What things do I need to know?

53 Introduction

54 **GH3.1** Prepare for hair services

54 Set up materials, tools and equipment

56 Make sure the stylist's tools are ready and safe to use

57 Get the client's records ready

58 **GH3.2** Maintain the work area for hair services

58 Dispose of waste materials

59 Check and clean the salon equipment

61 Prepare enough towels for the day

61 Refill and replenish low levels of salon stock

62 Replace the salon's resources correctly

63 Clean working surfaces properly so that they are ready for use

64 Checkerboard

64 Revision questions

Chapter**five**

65 **GH1 Shampoo and condition hair**

65 Unit GH1: quick overview

65 What do I need to do for GH1.1?

65 What do I need to do for GH1.2?

65 What do I need to do for GH1.3?

66 What things do I need to cover?

66 What things do I need to know?

66 Introduction

68 **GH1.1** Maintain effective and safe methods of working when shampooing and conditioning hair

68 Correctly protect and position clients and yourself

69 Keeping the basin area clean and safe to use

69 Maintaining personal hygiene standards

70 Monitoring the levels of materials

70 Completing the service efficiently

71 **GH1.2** Shampoo hair

71 Types of shampoo

72 Following the stylist's instructions

73 Using the correct massage techniques

75 Controlling the water flow and temperature

75 Rinsing and finishing off

76 **GH1.3** Apply conditioners to the hair

76 Following the stylist's instructions

76 Using the appropriate technique

78 Rinsing and finishing off

79 Checkerboard

79 Revision questions

Chapter**six**

80 **GH2 Blow dry hair**

80 Unit GH2: quick overview

80 What do I need to do for GH2.1?

80 What do I need to do for GH2.2?

80 What things do I need to cover?

81 What things do I need to know?

81 Introduction

82 **GH2.1** Maintain effective and safe methods of working when drying hair

82 Correctly protect and position clients and yourself

82 Keeping the work area clean and safe to use at all times

83 Maintaining personal hygiene standards

83 Using tools and resources safely

86 Completing the service efficiently

87 **GH2.2** Blow dry hair

87 Following the stylist's instructions

88 Applying the products correctly
90 Maintaining the client's comfort
90 Using brushes to style hair professionally
95 Checkerboard
95 Revision questions

Chapter**seven**

96 **GH4 Assist with hair colouring services**

96 Unit GH4: quick overview
96 What do I need to do for GH4.1?
96 What do I need to do for GH4.2?
96 What things do I need to cover?
97 What things do I need to know?
97 Introduction
97 **GH4.1 Maintain effective and safe methods of working when assisting with colouring services**

97 Learning why hair is different colours
98 Learning about colouring techniques
99 Correctly protect and position the client and yourself
100 Maintaining personal hygiene standards
100 Keeping the work area clean and safe to use at all times
101 Identifying when colours need reordering
101 **GH4.2 Remove colouring and lightening products**

101 Minimising the risk of hair damage
102 Keeping the client adequately protected
104 Applying suitable conditioners
105 Leaving the client ready for further services
105 Checkerboard
105 Revision questions

Chapter**eight**

106 **GH5 Assist with perming hair services**

106 Unit GH5: quick overview
106 What do I need to do for GH5.1?
106 What do I need to do for GH5.2?
106 What things do I need to know?
107 Introduction
107 **GH5.1 Maintain effective and safe methods of working when assisting with perming services**

108 Correctly protect and position the client and yourself
109 Keeping work areas clean and safe to use at all times
110 Maintaining personal hygiene standards
110 Reporting low neutralising products' stock
111 **GH5.2 Neutralise hair as part of the perming process**

111 Neutralising (rebalancing the hair)
112 Preparing the neutraliser properly

112 Rinsing perm lotion from hair properly
112 Applying the neutraliser correctly
113 Applying a suitable conditioner
115 Checkerboard
115 Revision questions

Chapter**nine**

116 **GH6 Plait and twist hair using basic techniques**

116 Unit GH6: quick overview
116 What do I need to do for GH6.1?
116 What do I need to do for GH6.2?
116 What things do I need to cover?
117 What things do I need to know?
117 Introduction
117 **GH6.1 Maintain effective and safe methods of working when plaiting and twisting**

118 Correctly protect and position clients and yourself
119 Keeping work areas clean at all times
119 Maintaining personal hygiene standards
120 Completing the service efficiently
120 **GH6.2 Plait and twist hair**

120 Preparing the client
121 Controlling your tools
121 Securing the free ends of plaits
122 Learning about hair textures
122 Maintaining an even tension
122 Applying suitable products
124 Checking clients' comfort and satisfaction
124 Creating loose hanging plaits
126 Making French plaits and twists
127 Applying twisting techniques
130 Checkerboard
130 Revision questions

Chapter**ten**

131 **GH7 Remove hair extensions**

131 Unit GH7: quick overview
131 What do I need to do for GH7.1?
131 What do I need to do for GH7.2?
131 What things do I need to cover?
132 What things do I need to know?
132 Introduction
135 **GH7.1 Maintain effective and safe methods of working when removing hair extensions**

135 Correctly protect and position clients and yourself
137 Keeping work areas clean at all times

137 Maintaining personal hygiene standards
137 Using tools and materials safely
139 **GH7.2 Remove hair extensions**
139 Listening to the stylist's instructions
139 Minimising the risk of hair damage
139 Ensuring that the client is comfortable
140 Preparing the hair for the service
140 Learning about removal techniques
143 Checkerboard
143 Revision questions

Chapter**eleven**

144 **GB1 Assist with shaving services**
144 Unit GB1: quick overview
144 What do I need to do for GB1.1?
144 What do I need to do for GB1.2?
144 What things do I need to cover?
145 What things do I need to know?
145 Introduction
146 **GB1.1 Maintain effective and safe methods of working when assisting with shaving services**

146 Correctly protect and position clients and yourself
147 Keeping work areas clean and safe to use at all times
148 Maintaining personal hygiene standards
148 Cleaning tools and equipment
151 Dealing with waste and shortages
152 Learning about shaving products
153 **GB1.2 Prepare facial hair and skin for shaving services**
153 Cleansing and exfoliating the skin
153 Applying hot and cold towels
154 Applying lathering products
155 Telling the barber when the client is prepared
155 Removing lather and cooling the skin
157 Checkerboard
157 Revision questions

158 Appendix 1 Health and safety legislation
162 Appendix 2 People's rights and consumer legislation
165 Answers to revision questions
166 Useful addresses and websites
168 Glossary
170 Index

Foreword

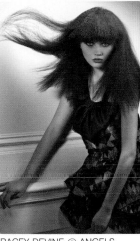

TRACEY DEVINE @ ANGELS

What do you want to do when you leave school? You probably want a role that is exciting, vibrant and varied which will lead to an interesting future.

Let Martin Green's *Begin Hairdressing & Barbering* inspire you to start your qualification in hairdressing, which will bring you a rewarding and fruitful career with endless prospects for future development. With over 30 years of practical experience, Martin is an accomplished professional whose wealth of experience, knowledge and understanding of the industry shine through in this informative and comprehensive book that will become an invaluable source of guidance as you start work.

The British hairdressing industry is renowned for having the highest standards in the world and with high standards comes hard work and a determination to meet the standards of the industry and of your clients. The reward is real satisfaction when you see the results of your work in your client's hair and the real motivator and testimony to your success is when your client's look and persona is transformed by your work.

It is also to Martin's credit that *Begin Hairdressing & Barbering* is now in its latest edition. I am delighted that Martin has actively and consistently updated the original book in keeping with changes, such as the introduction of the Qualifications and Credit Framework (QCF). You'll also find that *Begin Hairdressing & Barbering – The Official Guide to Level 1, Revised 2e* makes a great companion to some of the other learning resources available from Habia and Cengage Learning, such as our U2Learn online learning range, showing its versatility and worth to learners and educators alike.

I am incredibly proud of the association between Habia and the author of this book, and hope that for you this is the starting point to a long and successful career.

Alan Goldsbro
Chief Executive Officer
Habia

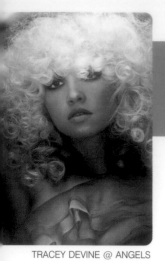
TRACEY DEVINE @ ANGELS

Acknowledgements

The authors and publishers would like to thank the following:

For providing pictures for the book

Adam Harris @ MG Martin Gold, Stanmore
Alamy
Andrew O'Toole (Photographer)
Anne McGuigan @ Anne McGuigan Hair and Beauty,
   Leighton Buzzard
BaByliss Pro
Balmain
Beauty Express
Ben White and the Eleven Hair Art Team
Christopher Appleton @ George's Hair Salon, Leicester
Chubb
Ciente @ Berkhamsted
Cinderella Hair (www.cinderellahair.co.uk)
Connect-2-Hair Ltd.
Corbis
Damien Carney for Joico
Daniele Cipriani (Photographer)
Denman
Dome Cosmetics
Ellisons
Errol Douglas
Essence PR
Fellowship for British Hairdressing F.A.M.E. Team 2008
Gloss Communications
Goldwell UK
Gorgeous PR
Great Lengths (www.greatlengths.net)
Habia
Hama Sanders (Photographer)
HMSO
i-salon
i-stock photography
Jemico
Karen Scantlebury @ Ciente, Berkhamsted
Karine Jackson Hair & Beauty

Ken Picton @ Ken Picton
Kiyoshi Inoue and Tim Hartley for DAVINES
Kyoko Homma (Photographer)
L. Professionnel
Lee Moran @ Sanrizz
Leonardo Rizzo @ Sanrizz
Lewis Moore @ Francesco Group, Streetly
Lynne Welsh @ Mosko, Wishaw
M. Balfre
Mahogany Hairdressing Salons and Academy
   (www.mahoganyhair.co.uk)
Mark Woolley (Hair stylist)
Matrix
Mediscan
Melanie Tudor@ En Route Hair and Beauty, Wakefield
Michael Barnes for Goldwell
NHF Inspire, Photography: Simon Powell
Ozzie Rizzo (Photography)
Paul Falltrick for Matrix
Paul Hawes @ Review, Petersfield and Waterlooville,
   Hants
Pete Webb (Photographer)
Pro Tip
Rae Palmer for Schwarzkopf
Reds Hair & Beauty, Sunderland
REM
Richard Ward
Route, Wakefield
Rush London
Saks Hair & Beauty (www.saks.co.uk)
SANRIZZ Artistic Team
Scott Smurthwaite @ Cream
Sharon Cox @ Sanrizz
Solara & Mantis
Sorisa
Susan Hall @ Reds Hair and Beauty, Sunderland

Terry Calvert and the Clipso Artistic Team
The Artistic Team @ Jacks of London
The John Rawson partnership
Theresa Bullock
Tim Lawton and The Artistic Team @ TPL Hairdressing,
    Nantwich
TPL Hairdressing, Crewe
Tracey Devine @ Angels, Aberdeen
UK Skills
Vicky Turner @ Goldsworthy's
Wahl (UK) Ltd
Wella

For their help with the photoshoot:
Hair: Patrick Cameron for Babyliss Pro; photography:
Thornton Howdle; make-up: Alison Chesterton; clothes:
Accent, Leeds

Photoshoot location:
HQ Hair
71 High Street, and 25 Cambray Place, Cheltenham Glos

Models:
Holly Batin
Alex Bilak
Dale Carney

Elisabeth Crabbe
Gareth Dazely
Lucy Dix
Jamie Horder
Sara Horder
Sian Jennings
Es John
Teyah Lee
Sean O'Riley
Tom O'Shea
Caroline Palmer
Laura Paoletti
Lucia Parry
Dawn Stanley

Stylists:
Becci Fincham
Jodi Green
Martin Green
HQ Hair Cheltenham

Make up:
Holly Batin

Photography:
Fi Deane

A special Thank You
Goldwell for all their help and support in providing the products and technical assistance within the photo shoot.

Every effort has been made to trace the copyright holders, but if any have been inadvertently overlooked the publisher will be pleased to make the necessary arrangements at the first opportunity. Please contact the publisher directly.

Introduction

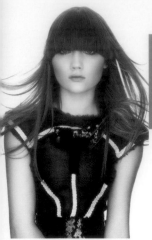

SCOTT SMURTHWAITE @ CREAM

Choices, choices. So many different occupations, so how do you choose?

It's very difficult knowing what you want to do when you haven't got anything to compare it against. You don't know what the work involves or whether you will like it. Well, this book will try to give you some help in at least one of those areas.

Hairdressing and barbering are and always has been a popular choice for many young people. Each year around twenty thousand people believe that that is the right choice for them and historically, the statistics tell us that most of those people decide to stay. From these figures, those students that have completed Level 1 say that they have enjoyed what they have learned and intend to use it as good preparation for a life-long career.

I wish you every success in hairdressing or barbering and hope it brings you as much pleasure and fulfilment as it has done for me.

Good luck

Martin Green

Qualification information

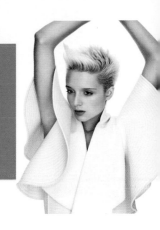

About the Level 1 NVQ Certificate in Hairdressing and Barbering

The structure of the qualification:

The Level 1 Certificate is made up from a total of 11 units. Some of these are compulsory, i.e. you have to do them, and the others leave you with choices or options. Quite simply, you choose the ones that interest you. This flexible arrangement means that you are in control of what you want to do.

So, looking at the structure of the full qualification a little more closely, we see that all students have to complete the **four mandatory units** and then choose other units that make up a **minimum of six optional credits**.

Mandatory units:

Unit:	Value
G20 Ensure responsibility for actions to reduce risks to health and safety (ENTO Unit HSS 1)	(4 credits)
G3 Contribute to the development of effective working relationships	(4 credits)
GH1 Shampoo and condition hair	(4 credits)
GH3 Prepare for hair services and maintain work areas	(2 credits)

(All must be completed.)

PLUS a minimum of **six optional credits** from the list below:

Unit:	Value
G2 Assist with salon reception duties	(4 credits)
GH2 Blow dry hair	(4 credits)
GH4 Assist with hair colouring services	(4 credits)
GH5 Assist with perming hair services	(3 credits)
GH6 Plait and twist hair using basic techniques	(4 credits)
GH7 Remove hair extensions	(3 credits)
GB1 Assist with shaving services	(2 credits)

Unit structure:

You can see that each unit has a title and this indicates the area of work that it involves. Within each unit there are a varying number of tasks that need to be performed and passed; in order to complete the whole unit.

A unit is the smallest component of the qualification that can be awarded. In other words, if someone didn't complete the full qualification, then they can get acknowledgement for those units that they did complete.

Let's take a closer look at what each of the mandatory and optional units comprise of.

We can now see for instance that Unit **GH3 Prepare for hairdressing services and maintain work areas** has a value of **four credits** and is made up from two main outcomes: **GH3.1 Prepare for salon services** and **GH3.2 Maintain the work area for hairdressing services.**

Unit	Main Outcomes
G20 Make sure your own actions reduce risks to health and safety **(4 credits)**	G20.1 Identify the hazards and evaluate the risks in your workplace G20.2 Reduce the risks to health and safety in your workplace
G3 Contribute to the development of effective working relationships **(4 credits)**	G3.1 Develop effective working relationships with clients G3.2 Develop effective working relationships with colleagues G3.3 Develop yourself within the job role
GH1 Shampoo and condition hair **(4 credits)**	GH1.1 Maintain effective and safe methods of working when shampooing and conditioning hair GH1.2 Shampoo hair GH1.2 Apply conditioners to the hair
GH3 Prepare for hairdressing services and maintain work areas **(2 credits)**	GH3.1 Prepare for salon services GH3.2 Maintain the work area for hairdressing services

We also know that to achieve a full qualification at Level 1 that a minimum of **six credits** must also be completed from the following units.

G2 Assist with salon reception duties **(4 credits)**	G2.1 Maintain the reception area G2.2 Attend to clients and enquiries G2.3 Help to make appointments for salon services
GH2 Blow dry hair **(4 credits)**	GH2.1 Maintain effective & safe methods of working when drying hair GH2.2 Blow dry hair
GH4 Assist with hair colouring services **(4 credits)**	GH4.1 Maintain effective and safe methods of working when assisting with colouring services GH4.2 Remove colouring and lightening products.
GH5 Assist with perming hair services **(3 credits)**	GH5.1 Maintain effective and safe methods of working when assisting with perming services GH2.2 Neutralise hair as part of the perming process

GH6 Plait and twist hair using basic techniques (4 credits)	GH6.1 Maintain effective and safe methods of working when plaiting and twisting GH6.2 Plait and twist hair
GH7 Remove hair extensions (3 credits)	GH7.1 Maintain effective and safe methods of working when removing hair extensions GH7.2 Remove hair extensions
GB1Assist with shaving services (2 credits)	GB1.1 Maintain effective and safe methods of working when assisting with shaving services GB1.2 Prepare facial hair and skin for shaving services

National Vocational Qualifications (NVQs)

You probably noticed that National Vocational Qualifications (NVQs) are set out in the same way. They all have:

- a unit title
- a unit reference number
- a credit value
- main outcomes.

This provides a simple, at-a-glance way of identifying the related tasks. However, it does not explain what you need to know, or what is required when you are being assessed.

To find this out, you need to know that each of the main outcomes are broken down into the following components:

1 **Performance criteria** – a list of statements that form a sort of checklist that describe how each task **must** be done.

2 **Range** – a variety of conditions, or situations, in which the task should be carried out.

3 **Knowledge and understanding** – a list of things that you **must** know that are essential to the task.

Example of performance criteria, range, knowledge and understanding

This is main outcome:

G3.1 Develop effective working relationships with clients

The performance criteria says what you have to do:

1 communicating with clients in a manner which promotes goodwill, trust and maintains confidentiality

2 handling client belongings with care and returning them when required

3 promptly referring any client concerns to the relevant person

4 maintaining client comfort and care to the satisfaction of the client

5 meeting your salon's standards for appearance and behaviour

The range says what you must cover:

1 active participation in training and development activities

2 active participation in salon activities

3 watching technical activities

The knowledge and understanding tells us what we need to know

1 how to communicate in a clear, polite, confident way and why this is important

2 the questioning and listening skills you need in order to find out information

3 the rules and procedures regarding the methods of communication you use

4 how to recognise when a client is angry and when a client is confused

Completing the activities

All the essential parts of your Level 1 qualification can be found within the chapters of this book. Within each chapter you will find a variety of activities that will help you to learn the things that you need to know.

By doing these activities you can:

- make it easier to remember all the important information
- make better preparations for your assessments
- use the information that you create to provide supporting evidence for your portfolio.

Not all the activities can be answered from the information in this book. Many of them will need you to search for the answers in other places. This kind of private study or 'self-directed' learning will make it easier to remember the information at assessment time. As you work through this book, try to get into the habit of writing down important words. At the end of each chapter, make notes about the key facts and things that you have learnt.

Under assessment

Your ability to carry out a task to standard is measured during assessment. You will be observed and measured against the performance criteria from the National Occupational Standards (NOS). Sometimes, when it's not possible to cover all the situations that might crop up, your assessor might ask you questions about what you have done and how you might do something differently in a another situation. To help you get used to this, the activities sections contain lots of the types of questions that you might be asked.

Your knowledge and understanding of the different tasks are also assessed by question-and-answer techniques. Sometimes this could be in the form of written questions, like a multiple-choice quiz, or you might be asked to give a short description. In other situations you may just be asked questions orally, or your work or responses could be recorded on video. In either event, the activities in this book give you plenty of examples and practice.

About the book

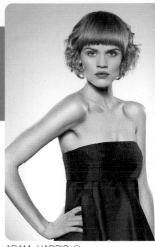

ADAM HARRIS @
MG MARTIN GOLD

The common structure and design that exist within NVQ Certificate are mirrored in many ways within this text. For the first time in the Level 1 NVQ Certificate in Hairdressing & Barbering official series, revisions and updates have been totally reworked to provide:

A the fastest possible navigation to the things that you want to find out about

B a book that covers all the aspects of the NVQ for both hairdressing and barbering standards

C a chapter structure that now mirrors the NVQ standards in unit as well as outcome format.

You will be able to navigate standards; getting faster access to the information and the unique EKU referencing system directs you straight to the information that you need to know.

All of these features and illustrations have been redesigned and reorganised in order to help you accelerate through your Level 1 programme.

How to use this book

You can use this book in a number of ways:

1 You can use the EKU reference map to quickly find text that covers the things that you want to know without having to wade through pages of text.

2 You can use the revised chapter structure to cover complete units as you get to them within your training.

3 You can use the book as a quick guide and overview to the things that you will be doing and the things that you will learn.

4 You can use it as your standalone course guide covering the A–Z of hairdressing and barbering at Level 1.

This new format will help you to use and read this book more easily. Each chapter addresses specific units from the NVQ/SVQ Level 1. At the beginning of each chapter a referencing system provides a quick signposting to the information you want, providing a variety of starting and finishing points. In this next example, you can see the variety of features and icons used within the text.

e-teaching website

A new **e-teaching website** for trainers accompaines this text book.

This resource includes **handouts, PowerPoint™ slides, interactive quizzes, an image bank** and **videoclips** – all carefully designed to help trainers make classroom delivery more interactive and to provide extra materials for lesson planning.

Please visit www.eteachhairdressing.co.uk for more information or contact your Cengage Learning sales representative at emea.fesales@cengage.com

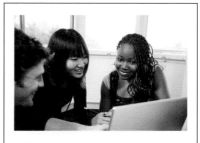

Learners!

Access your FREE online resources by following the Level 1 student links on www.eteachhairdressing .co.uk and entering your password 'fringe'

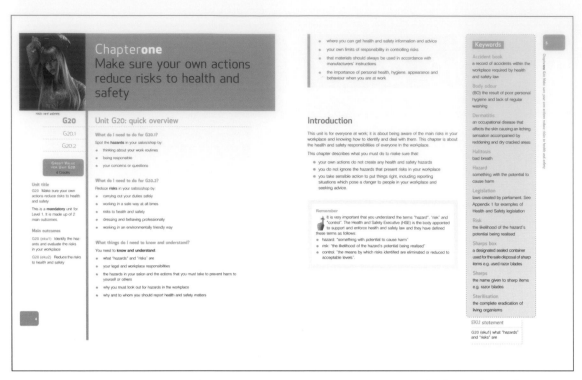

NVQ/reference, unit title and main outcome An at-a-glance overview of the unit and main outcomes covered in the chapter.

What do I need to do? A brief overview of the activities involved in the unit and customised information telling you what you need to do about practical tasks.

What do I need to cover? A quick guide that covers therange of things that are included and the contexts in whichthings will need to be done.

What do I need to know? Costomised information on what you need to learn and understand in order to complete a task satisfactorily.

Information covered in this chapter A list of information coveredwithin the chapter.

Key words Special or technical terms.

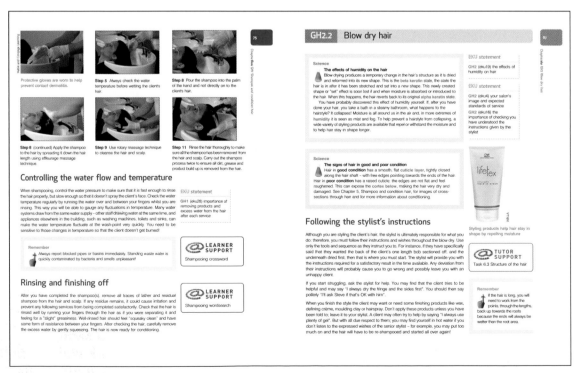

Step-by-steps Photo sequences to illustrate procedures.

Hair science Scientific principles that relate to hairdressing and barbering.

Learner support signposts Online activities available on the learner side of the eteachhairdressing website.

Tutor support signposts Online activities available on the tutor side of the eteachhairdressing website.

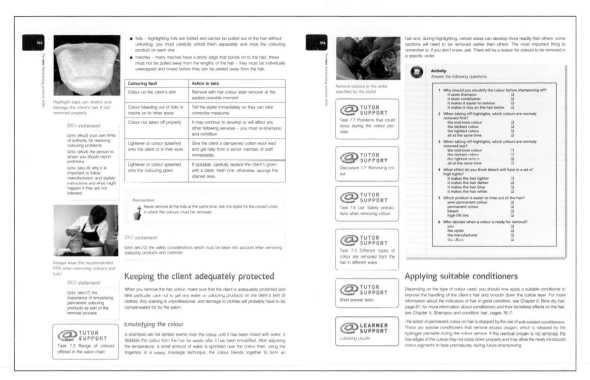

Remember boxes Tips or hints on points to remember.

EKU reference points These map the essential knowledge-required in the NOS standards directly to paragraphs covering this information.

Activities Placed throughout the book to give you practical-experience of things that you need to learn.

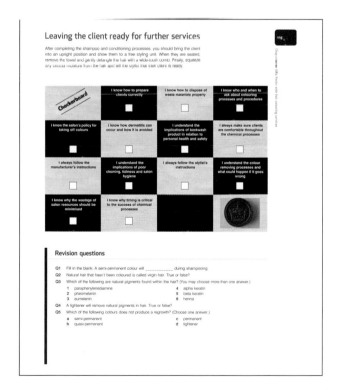

Checkerboard A self check system and means of recording progress towards achievement.

Tests A variety of self-assessment tests are available at the end of the chapter with answers at the back of the book.

EKU mapping grids

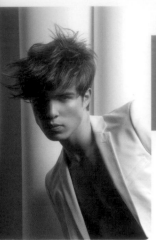

LEONARDO RIZZO @ SANRIZZ

To use these essential knowledge lookup tables, simply find the EKU statement in the NVQ Level 1 standards that you want to learn more about. Then using this grid match the number to its corresponding page.

For example, say that you want to look up the knowledge relating to: **G3.10 How to recognise when a client is angry and when a client is confused,** which is part of **Unit G3 Contribute to the development of effective working relationships.** Just look in the table G3 below and look at the corresponding page for EKU number 10.

Chapter**one**

G20 Make sure your own actions reduce risks to health and safety																		
EKU	1	2	3	4	5	6	7	8	9	10	11	12	13	14	15	16	17	
Page	5	7	7	7	7	7	8	8	10	8	18	8	7	10	19	20	11	

Chapter**two**

G3 Contribute to the development of effective working relationships																		
EKU	1	2	3	4	5	6	7	8	9	**10**	11	12	13	14	15	16	17	18	19
Page	33	29	29	29	29	24	24	24	32	**26**	33	34	33	33	31	31	31	32	32
EKU	20	21	22	23	24														
Page	32	29	33	30	29														

Chapter**three**

G2 Assist with salon reception duties																		
EKU	1	2	3	4	5	6	7	8	9	10	11	12	13	14	15	16	17	18	19
Page	40	38	44	41	48	44	43	38	41	41	41	41	41	42	46	42	42	38	46

Chapter**four**

GH3 Prepare for hair services and maintain work areas																		
EKU	1	2	3	4	5	6	7	8	9	10	11	12	13	14	15	16	17		
Page	54	57	62	54	57	57	57	56	54	53	56	62	56	57	59	59	62		

Chapter**five**

GH1 Shampoo and condition hair																		
EKU	1	2	3	4	5	6	7	8	9	10	11	12	13	14	15	16	17	18	19
Page	68	70	70	68	72	69	68	68	68	69	69	69	70	77	74	67	67	76	70
EKU	20	21	22	23	24	25	26	27	28	29	30	31							
Page	72	70	70	72	70	74	74	76	75	76	72	70							

Chapter**six**

GH2 Blow dry hair																		
EKU	1	2	3	4	5	6	7	8	9	10	11	12	13	14	15	16	17	18	19
Page	82	86	82	82	82	82	82	83	82	83	83	83	83	83	83	87	90	92	87
EKU	20	21	22	23	24	25	26												
Page	92	91	83	88	91	92	92												

Chapter**seven**

GH4 Assist with hair colouring services																		
EKU	1	2	3	4	5	6	7	8	9	10	11	12	13	14	15	16	17	18	19
Page	97	97	102	102	100	100	99	99	100	100	100	102	100	100	101	101	102	99	102
EKU	20																		
Page	101																		

Chapter**eight**

GH5 Assist with perming hair services																		
EKU	1	2	3	4	5	6	7	8	9	10	11	12	13	14	15	16	17	18	19
Page	108	109	111	110	109	110	108	108	108	110	109	108	109	110	110	107	111	111	109
EKU	20	21	22																
Page	111	113	113																

Chapter**nine**

GH6 Plait and twist hair using basic techniques																		
EKU	1	2	3	4	5	6	7	8	9	10	11	12	13	14	15	16	17	18	19
Page	119	119	120	119	119	119	119	119	119	119	120	120	121	120	124	124	124	119	121
EKU	20	21	22	23	24	25	26												
Page	125	122	121	122	122	122	122												

Chapter**ten**

GH7 Remove hair extensions																			
EKU	1	2	3	4	5	6	7	8	9	10	11	12	13	14	15	16	17	18	19
Page	135	135	135	135	136	135	135	135	135	135	135	137	137	137	137	137	139	139	139
EKU	20	21	22	23	24	25	26												
Page	134	139	139	134	140	140	137												

Chapter**eleven**

GB1 Assist with shaving services																			
EKU	1	2	3	4	5	6	7	8	9	10	11	12	13	14	15	16	17	18	19
Page	146	151	151	148	146	146	146	146	146	147	146	152	147	151	148	148	152	152	154
EKU	20	21	22	23	24	25	26												
Page	153	151	151	155	156	154	155												

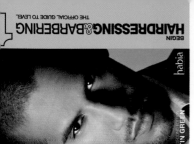

BEGIN HAIRDRESSING & BARBERING
VRQ mapping grid

Unit Ref	Unit credit (QCF)	VRQ Unit Title	Unit Level	Ch1 G20	Ch2 G3	Ch3 G2	Ch4 GH3	Ch5 GH1	Ch6 GH2	Ch7 GH4	Ch8 GH5	Ch9 GH6	Ch10 GH7	Ch11 GB1
F/502/3846	2	Present a professional image	1	X	X									
M/502/3759	3	Introduction to Basic styling for women?	1						X					
H/502/3760	3	Introduction to Basic styling for men?	1						X					
Y/502/3805	3	Introduction to plaiting and twisting	1									X		
R/600/6334	3	Salon reception duties	1		X									
H/600/6323	2	Working with others in a salon	1		X									
Y/600/6335	2	Create and maintain retail displays in a salon	1			X								
A/600/6327	3	Follow health and safety in the salon	1	X										
Y/600/4875	3	Create a hair and beauty image	1											
R/600/4874	1	Colour hair using temporary colour	1							X				
A/502/3795	3	Styling Men's Hair	1						X					

Hairdressing
E-Teaching Website

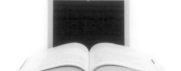

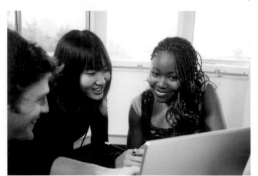

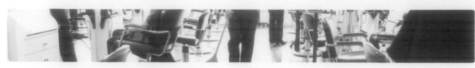

e-teaching website

A **new e-teaching website** for trainers accompanies this text book.

This resource includes **handouts, PowerPoint™ slides, interactive quizzes,** an **image bank** and **videoclips** – all carefully designed to help trainers make classroom delivery more interactive and to provide extra materials for lesson planning.

Please visit www.eteachhairdressing.co.uk for more information or contact your Cengage Learning sales representative at emea.fesales@cengage.com.

Students! Access your FREE online resources by following the Level 1 student links on www.eteachhairdressing.co.uk and entering your password 'fringe'.

TUTOR SUPPORT

Links to the e-teach resources are flagged throughout the text. If your trainer subscribes to one e-teaching website, they will be able to download these and use them in class.

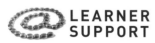

LEARNER SUPPORT

Free online student resources are available wherever you see this red symbol.

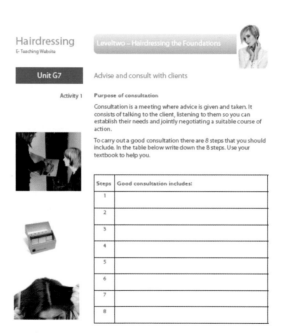

Hairdressing
E-Teaching Website

Leveltwo – Hairdressing the Foundations

Unit G7   Advise and consult with clients

Activity 1   **Purpose of consultation**

Consultation is a meeting where advice is given and taken. It consists of talking to the client, listening to them so you can establish their needs and jointly negotiating a suitable course of action.

To carry out a good consultation there are 8 steps that you should include. In the table below write down the 8 steps. Use your textbook to help you.

Steps	Good consultation includes:
1	
2	
3	
4	
5	
6	
7	
8	

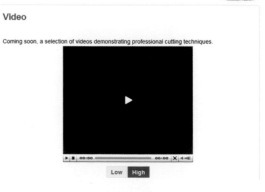

Hairdressing
E-Teaching Website

Leveltwo - Hairdressing the Foundations
Logged in as lucy mills (logout)   Change level:

Level 2 contents		
Units		
G8	G4	G7
GH12	AH21	GH9/GB2
Gen 1	Gen 2	Gen 3
Gen 4		

Key Teaching Strategies
Glossary
Feedback
Useful weblinks
Fun weblinks

Video

Coming soon, a selection of videos demonstrating professional cutting techniques.

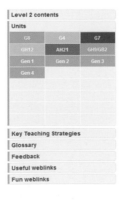

Low   High

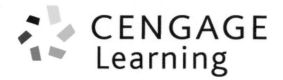 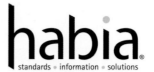

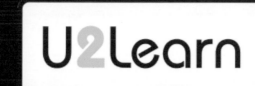

ONLINE LEARNING RESOURCES
FOR HAIRDRESSERS AND BEAUTY THERAPISTS

Produced in partnership by Cengage Learning and Habia, U2Learn is a ground-breaking e-learning solution for Beauty Therapy and Hairdressing students. Available online to provide qualification coverage in class, in the salon or at home. U2Learn is interactive and fun for you and your learners and offers a wealth of video clips, animations and activities to bring learning to life! Each U2Learn product offers you flexibility in your purchasing and can be bought as a complete package or per module.

For more information about our U2Learn solution, contact our sales team at emea_fesales@cengage.com

U2Learn Hairdressing

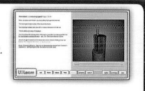

U2Learn Hairdressing offers a one-stop-shop e-learning solution for Hairdressing at Level 2.

U2Learn Hairdressing can be purchased **per module** or as a **whole package**:

The modules within U2Learn Hairdressing are:

- Salon legislation
- Salon reception
- Selling skills
- Consultation
- Positive effectiveness
- Cut hair

- Shampoo, condition and treat the hair and scalp
- Style and set hair
- Perm and neutralise hair
- Colour hair
- Plait and twist hair – Coming soon!
- Attach hair to enhance a style – Coming soon!

U2Learn Hairdressing is the perfect partner to *Palladino's Hairdressing: The Foundations - The Official Guide to Hairdressing Level 2* textbook, but can also be used as a stand-alone teaching and learning resource.

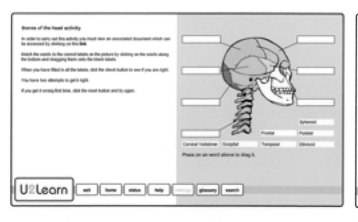

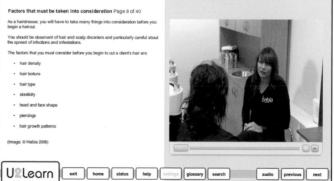

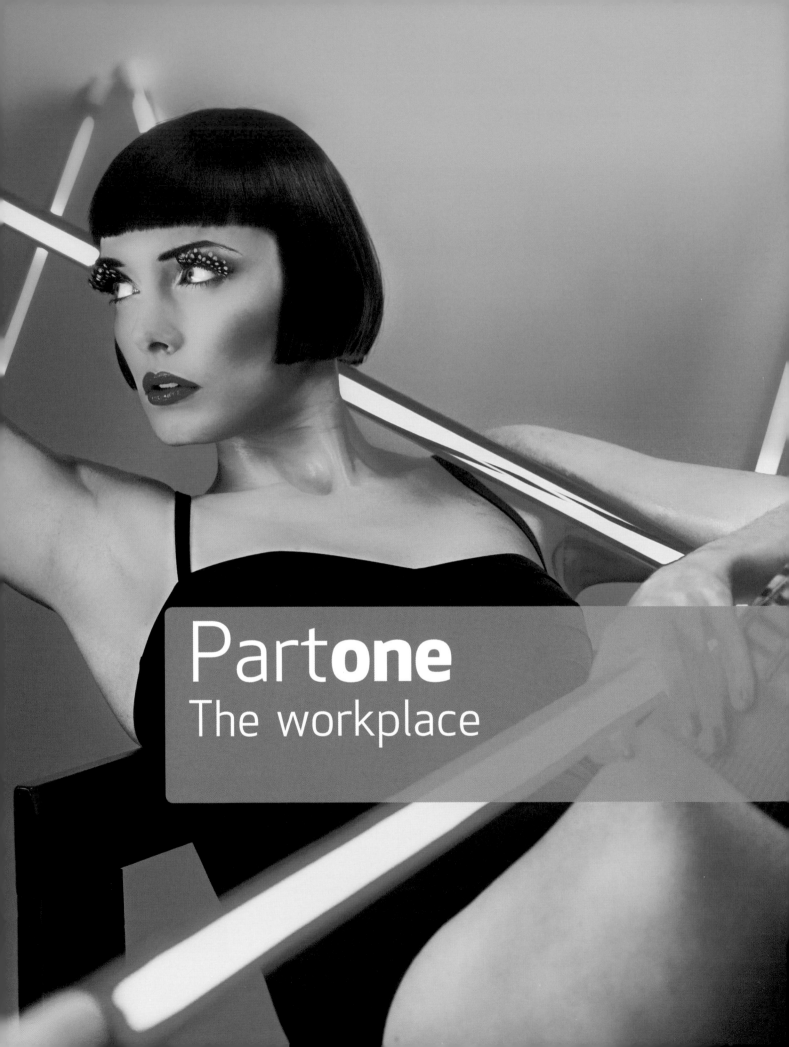

Part**one**
The workplace

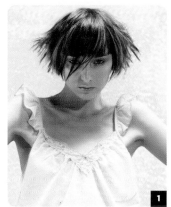

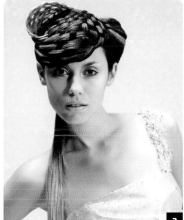

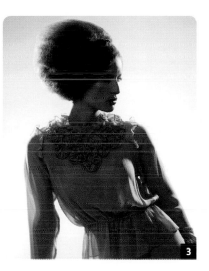

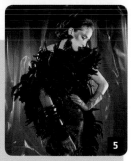

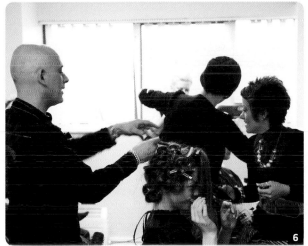

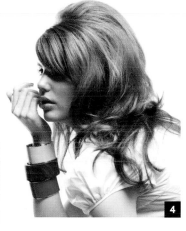

1 Vicky Turner @ Goldsworthy's 2 Vicky Turner @ Goldsworthy's 3 Ken Picton @ Ken Picton 4 Paul Hawes @ Review, Petersfield and Waterlooville, Hants 5 Hair: Richard Ward, Photography: Daniele Cipriani 6 Hair: NHF Inspire, Photography: Simon Powell **Left** Sanrizz Spectrum Collection by Sanrizz Artistic Team

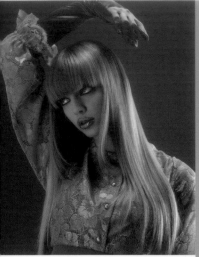

Chapter**one**
Make sure your own actions reduce risks to health and safety

G20

G20.1

G20.2

**CREDIT VALUE
FOR UNIT G20**
4 Credits

Unit title

G20 Make sure your own actions reduce risks to health and safety

This is a **mandatory** unit for Level 1. It is made up of 2 main outcomes.

Main outcomes

G20 (eku1) Identify the hazards and evaluate the risks in your workplace

G20 (eku2) Reduce the risks to health and safety

Unit G20: quick overview

What do I need to do for G20.1?

Spot the **hazards** in your salon/shop by:

- thinking about your work routines
- being responsible
- your concerns or questions

What do I need to do for G20.2?

Reduce **risks** in your salon/shop by:

- carrying out your duties safely
- working in a safe way at all times
- risks to health and safety
- dressing and behaving professionally
- working in an environmentally friendly way

What things do I need to know and understand?

You need to **know and understand**:

- what "hazards" and "risks" are
- your legal and workplace responsibilities
- the hazards in your salon and the actions that you must take to prevent harm to yourself or others
- why you must look out for hazards in the workplace
- why and to whom you should report health and safety matters

- where you can get health and safety information and advice
- your own limits of responsibility in controlling risks
- that materials should always be used in accordance with manufacturers' instructions
- the importance of personal health, hygiene, appearance and behaviour when you are at work

Introduction

This unit is for everyone at work; it is about being aware of the main risks in your workplace and knowing how to identify and deal with them. This chapter is about the health and safety responsibilities of everyone in the workplace.

This chapter describes what you must do to make sure that:

- your own actions do not create any health and safety hazards
- you do not ignore the hazards that present risks in your workplace
- you take sensible action to put things right, including reporting situations which pose a danger to people in your workplace and seeking advice.

Remember

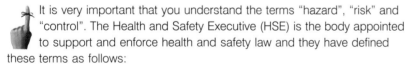 It is very important that you understand the terms "hazard", "risk" and "control". The Health and Safety Executive (HSE) is the body appointed to support and enforce health and safety law and they have defined these terms as follows:

- hazard: "something with potential to cause harm"
- risk: "the likelihood of the hazard's potential being realised"
- control: "the means by which risks identified are eliminated or reduced to acceptable levels".

G20.1 Identify the hazards and evaluate the risks in your workplace

TUTOR SUPPORT

Activity 1.1 Identify hazards and evaluate the risks in your workplace

TUTOR SUPPORT

Task 1.1 Potential hazards

TUTOR SUPPORT

Task 1.3 Health and safety regulations chart

Almost anything may be a hazard, but may or may not become a risk. The following are typical examples of hazards which present the highest risks in a salon or barber's shop:

1 A trailing electric cable from a piece of equipment is a hazard. If it is trailing across a passageway there is a high risk of someone tripping over it, but if it lies along a wall out of the way, the risk is much less.

2 Poisonous or flammable chemicals are hazards and may present a high risk. However, if they are kept in a properly designed secure store and handled by properly trained and equipped people, the risk is much less than if they are left about for anyone to use or misuse.

3 A failed light bulb is a hazard. If it is just one bulb out of many in a room it presents very little risk, but if it is the only light on a stairwell, it is a very high risk. Changing the bulb may be a high risk, if it is high up, or if the power has been left on, or low risk if it is in a table lamp which has been unplugged.

4 A box of heavy material is a hazard. It presents a higher risk to someone who lifts it incorrectly, rather than someone who uses the correct manual handling techniques.

Activity

Think about some of the hazards that could exist in your workplace. Now look at the table below and fill in the missing information.

Potential hazard	Why is this a hazard in the salon/shop?	How could this risk be reduced?
loose carpet edge in reception		
boxes stacked up in the fire escape		
water spilt on the floor near the basins		
hair clippings left on the salon floor		
loose plug on a blow dryer		
a stylist drops their comb on the floor, picks it up and then uses it on a client		

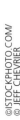

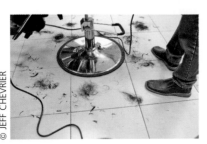

Hair clippings are an environmental hazard

You must be aware of the following categories of hazards in the workplace:

1 Hazards to do with the **environment** such as:

- wet or slippery floors
- cluttered passageways or corridors
- hair clippings left on the salon floor
- trailing electrical flexes.

2 Hazards to do with **equipment and materials**, such as:

- worn or faulty electrical equipment
- incorrectly labelled materials
- mishandling or inaccurate measurement of chemicals.

3 Hazards connected with **people**, such as:

- bad posture
- handling and moving stock
- poor health, cross-infection, disease.

Thinking about your work routines

You must identify the working practices which could harm yourself or other people. You work with others in a service for the public, so **all** of your day-to-day routines will have some form of impact on someone else. You have to keep and remain alert at all times when you are working. Legally, you have a duty of care not only to yourself, but also anyone else who could be affected by your actions. Your physical wellbeing is vitally important. Too many late nights and over-indulgences such as food and alcohol or added stress from personal issues will affect the way that you carry out your duties. Any lapses in your concentration or focus can have a disastrous impact on you, your work colleagues, or any of the salon's clients or visitors.

Activity

Think about the jobs that you do on a daily basis. What sorts of things could go wrong if you had a lapse in your concentration? Fill in the table below to identify the sorts of things that could happen and what you could do to rectify the situation.

Area of work	What could go wrong?	What should you do?
applying a neutraliser to curlers on a client		
taking a colour off at the basin		
mixing up a colour for a stylist, but use the wrong hydrogen peroxide		
a large delivery of stock arrives at reception and you move it to the stock room		
preparing a styling unit with equipment for a stylist, but a lead is loose on a blow dryer		

Being responsible

Simply being aware of potential hazards is not enough. You have a responsibility to contribute to a safe working environment, so you must take steps to check and deal with any sources of risk.

Suppose, for example, that someone had carelessly blocked a fire door with recently delivered stock. You could take the initiative and move the stock items to a safe and secure location. Or suppose you notice that someone else has left a saucepan of soup on the gas hob and has been called away to shampoo. You would turn the gas off and

EKU *statement*

G20 (eku3) your responsibilities for health and safety as required by the law covering your job role

Remember

Employers have a responsibility to ensure the health, safety and welfare of the people within the workplace. All people at work have a duty and responsibility not to harm themselves or others through the work they do.

EKU *statement*

G20 (eku2) your responsibilities and legal duties for health and safety in the workplace

G20 (eku4) the hazards which exist in your workplace and the safe working practices which you must follow

G20 (eku5) the particular health and safety hazards which may be present in your own job and the precautions you must take

G20 (eku6) the importance of remaining alert to the presence of hazards in the whole workplace

G20 (eku13) workplace instructions for managing risks which you are unable to deal with

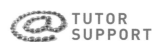

TUTOR SUPPORT

Task 1.2 Health and safety responsibility in the salon

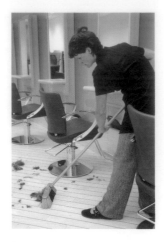

Sweep the floor to remove the hazard of hair clippings

EKU *statement*

G20 (eku7) the importance of dealing with, or promptly reporting, risks

G20 (eku10) the responsible people you should report health and safety matters to

Remember

 Being aware of potential hazards is not enough: minimise risks by taking prompt action.

Remember

 Health and safety laws are being continually reviewed and updated. Make sure you are aware of the latest information and look at the health and safety posters within your salon.

EKU *statement*

G20 (eku8) the responsibilities for health and safety in your job description

G20 (eku12) your scope and responsibility for controlling risks

let them continue when they have finished. You can:

1 Deal directly with the hazard, which means that you have taken individual responsibility. This will probably apply to obvious hazards such as:

- trailing flexes – roll them up and store them safely
- cluttered doorways and corridors – remove objects and store them safely or dispose of them appropriately
- sweep the floor to remove loose hair clippings.

Your concerns or questions

There are occasions where being responsible requires that you make a quick judgement of what you have found and tell someone else. When you notice a potential hazard that you cannot easily rectify yourself, tell your supervisor immediately.

Imagine for a moment that the lower, cutting blade on a pair of clippers became loose. If this was unnoticed by one of the stylists they might pick the clippers up and use them on a client! Here, your swift action may save a client from a serious injury. You see the hazard and understand the risk, but leave the essential re-adjustment of the blades to a suitably trained person. You can:

2 Inform a responsible person, e.g. your manager or supervisor, of the hazard, which means that it becomes an organisational responsibility. This applies to hazards which are beyond your responsibility to deal with, such as:

- faulty equipment such as dryers, tongs, straightening irons, kettles, computers etc.
- worn floor coverings or broken tiles
- loose or damaged fittings, such as mirrors, shelves or back washes
- obstructions that are too heavy for you to move safely
- fire – follow the correct procedures to raise the alarm and help with the salon's evacuation procedures.

Activity

Find out the following information from your place of work and then copy the complete table in your portfolio for future reference.

Q. Who has overall responsibility for health and safety?

A. Name

Q. What is this person's role in the workplace?

A. Job role

Q. If you found something that you felt was not safe at work, who would you report to?

A. Name

Q. What sort of unsafe things do you think you might find? (List as many as you can.)

A.

Q. In relation to product use, why are manufacturers' instructions important?

A.

Q. What is the salon's policy in respect to maintaining a healthy and safe work environment?

A.

Carrying out your duties safely

Hair salons and barber's shops vary in size, location, layout and staffing, and this creates a unique set of needs for each work environment. Each business has its own set of rules relating to health and safety practices and this information is made known to you at the point you become employed – usually during your induction. Your induction training sets out the basic rules of your employment: what's expected of you and what you can expect from the company. During this preliminary training you may be given a lot of information for the future. Amongst this information will be the salon's policy in relation to the following health and safety issues:

- fire and emergency evacuation procedures
- people to whom you should report to in the event of emergency or significant risk to people's safety
- the things that you **may** and **may not** undertake yourself to control risks to the health, safety and welfare of others
- health and safety training information.

In addition to the above, you will find the following prominently placed health and safety notices/records, available on display.

- health and safety law poster
- **COSHH** information booklet
- salon **risk assessment**
- Public Liability Insurance certificate
- fire safety evacuation procedures
- **accident book** (records of injuries and treatments provided)
- written health and safety policy (in work locations with more than 5 employees).

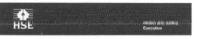

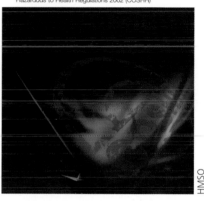

COSHH: A brief guide to the Regulations
What you need to know about the Control of Substances Hazardous to Health Regulations 2002 (COSHH)

HMSO

The HSE provides guidance on COSHH

EKU *statement*

G20 (eku2) your responsibilities and legal duties for health and safety in the workplace

Activity
Salon layout
Draw a floor plan of your salon. Show where the following can be found:

1 Fire extinguisher(s)

2 Storage for products/equipment

3 Disposal of waste and sharps.

4 Sterilising equipment

5 Personal protective equipment (PPE)

6 Accident book

7 Fire exit(s)

8 First aid box/kit

9 Health and safety information

10 Assembly point

Remember

We all have a duty to
safeguard the
environment that we
share. Be environmentally
friendly and aware when you
dispose of waste.

The **Health and Safety at Work Act (HASAWA) 1974** is the main, over-arching legislation, made by parliament, relating to business premises, under which, all other regulations exist. Although the Act contains many individual regulations the responsibility for
maintaining these falls upon you and your employer. Employers have a legal duty to
ensure that:

- the premises are safe to work within
- all equipment and salon systems are safe to use
- employees have access to personal protective equipment
- health and safety systems are appropriately reviewed and updated
- train their staff so they can do their duties safely.

Employees have a legal duty to:

- follow appropriate systems of work laid down for their safety
- make proper use of equipment provided for their safety
- co-operate with their employer on health and safety matters
- inform the employer if they identify hazardous activities/situations
- take care to ensure that their activities do not put others at risk.

For more specific information on individual health and safety regulations, see Appendix 1.

Activity

The Health and Safety at Work Act 1974 is continually being reviewed and updated. It covers many smaller
component regulations. See if you can match the individual legal regulations on the left with the appropriate health
and safety issues on the right. (Tip: look at the regulation wording to work out its appropriate link.)

Workplace (Health, Safety and Welfare) Regulations 1992	always wear gloves and aprons when handling chemical compounds
Manual Handling Operations Regulations 1992	correct and safe operation of salon equipment
Provision and Use of Work Equipment Regulations (PUWER) 1998	salon chemical products must be stored and be kept safely at all times
Personal Protective Equipment at Work Regulations 1992	dermatitis is a notifiable skin condition that results from sensitivity to chemicals
Control of Substances Hazardous to Health (COSHH) Regulations 2002	monitoring and maintenance of workplace hygiene and cleanliness
Electricity at Work Regulations 1989	always keep well stocked, just in case of accidents occurring at work
Reporting of Injuries, Diseases and Dangerous Occurrences Regulations (RIDDOR) 1995	manufacturers' information relating to the use of chemical products
Cosmetic Products (Safety) Regulations 1989	the movement and handling of objects needs to be done safely and properly
Health and Safety (First Aid) Regulations 1981	items of salon electrical equipment must be checked and tested each year

Working in a safe way at all times

Passageways and corridors are dangerous, regardless of whether the obstruction is in doorways or a corridor, on stairs or in a fire exit. In an emergency, people might have to leave the salon in a hurry – perhaps even in the dark if the electricity has gone off.

- always be on the lookout for any obstruction in these areas
- if you see something that could present a risk, tell your work supervisor.

Disposal of waste

General waste Much of the waste produced in a salon or barber's shop is harmless, and as long as it has been placed in a strong polythene bin liner and tied at the top, it can be disposed of as general rubbish. Some items should be cleared away promptly or handled and disposed of with care. For example, simple hair clippings left on the salon floor are a potential hazard, although they would not be considered hazardous waste. They become a risk to health and safety when they are left on the salon floor. There they could easily be slipped on if they are not swept away immediately.

Everyday waste items such as empty polythene containers, cotton neck wool, end papers, packaging, etc. should be placed into bin liners/salon bins. When they are almost full, the polythene bin liners can be removed and sealed by tying in a knot. The empty swing bin should be washed with detergent, dried and a new bin liner installed.

Being environmentally aware requires us to be more responsible in the ways in which we dispose of our waste items. Different local authorities have specific arrangements for safe disposal and recycling.

Activity
Find out what the local arrangements are for each of the following items:

- aluminium foil and cans, glass bottles and plastic waste, packaging
- paper, cardboard and other biodegradables
- chemical hairdressing products in relation to disposal down drains
- aerosols and other pressurised items
- sharps.

Disposal of sharp items Sharp items such as disposable razor blades need to be handled with extreme care. Used **sharps** (the term used to describe them) must be disposed of carefully to prevent any injury or cross-infection. Razor blades and similar items should be placed into a **sharps box**: a safe, sealed container. When the container is full it can be disposed of safely. This type of salon waste should be kept away from general salon waste as special arrangements may be provided by your local authority.

Lifting and handling

Manual handling is an everyday part of salon processes and because of this, it is easy to sustain personal injury. Bad posture and incorrect handling of large and/or heavy items

EKU *statement*

G20 (eku17) the risks to the environment which may be present in your workplace and/or in your own job

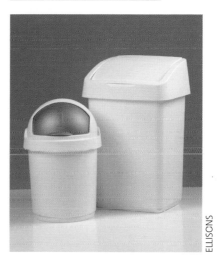

ELLISONS

An swing bin is acceptable for disposal of everyday waste

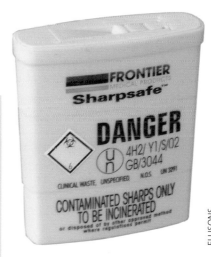

ELLISONS

Check with your local authority for requirements on disposal of sharps

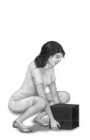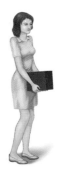

This shows the correct way to bend the knees when lifting awkward shapes

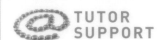

TUTOR SUPPORT

Activity 1.5 Fill in the gaps: Health and safety legislation

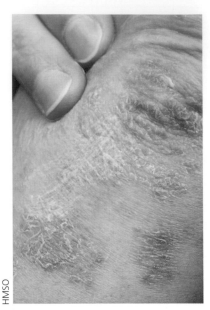

Dermatitis

Remember

Up to 70% of hairdressers suffer from skin damage. Keep your hands healthy and wave goodbye to bad hand days. Moisturise regularly and always wear disposable non-latex gloves when you handle any chemical products.

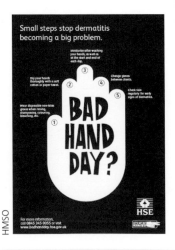

can result in low back pain/problems and strain disorders. Think about the situations that can occur in a salon environment, for example:

- moving stock into storage
- unpacking heavy or awkward items
- lifting equipment and moving salon furniture.

For more information on the Manual Handling Operations Regulations 1992, see Appendix 1.

Avoiding dermatitis

Many hairdressers have to give up hairdressing because of **dermatitis**. However, you can avoid this condition by making sure that you always use disposable vinyl gloves. Always dry your hands thoroughly after and moisturise to keep your hands healthy.

Five steps to preventing dermatitis

1 Wear disposable vinyl gloves when rinsing, shampooing, colouring, bleaching, etc.
2 Dry your hands thoroughly with a soft cotton or paper towel.
3 Moisturise after washing your hands, as well as at the start and end of each day. It's easy to miss fingertips, finger webs and wrists.
4 Change gloves between clients. Make sure you don't contaminate your hands when you take them off.
5 Check skin regularly for early signs of dermatitis.

What do you do if you think you have dermatitis? If you think you are suffering from dermatitis, visit your doctor for advice and treatment. If you believe it has been caused or made worse by your work as a trainee hairdresser/barber, mention this to your doctor and you must also tell your employer. They are required by law to report a case of work-related dermatitis amongst their staff.

Handling chemicals

Many hairdressing services involve some contact with chemicals, and you must always follow the product manufacturer's instructions for their safe use and application. Chemicals including perming lotions, neutralisers, colouring products and hydrogen peroxide are hazardous and present a high risk to anyone who does not handle them in the correct way. They must be handled, stored, used and disposed of correctly in accordance of the Control of Substances Hazardous to Health Regulations (2003), also known as the "COSHH Regulations". This means that every chemical product within the salon must be assessed for risk.

COSHH precautions Risk assessments are made by your employer. These will indicate the types of chemicals available within the salon and the safe ways in which they may be handled or used. The chemical products will vary from cleaning items (such as washing materials, bleach and polish), to the more typical salon specific items such as (colours, lighteners, hydrogen peroxide and general styling materials). Make sure that you use the lists provided by your employer. These will indicate:

- a hazard rating for each – the level of risk that each of the chemical products presents to you
- details on how they can be handled safely with the personal protective equipment (also known as "PPE").

See Appendix 1 for more information on the Personal Protective Equipment at Work Regulations 1992.

Equipment provided by your employer (PPE) Your employer provides PPE for you and the clients. Your protective equipment will be in the form of non-latex disposable gloves and plastic aprons; you **must** wear these items whenever you are handling chemicals. Watch the stylists to see the times when and the reasons why they wear these items.

The PPE for clients are gowns, towels and plastic capes. Clients should wear the sleeved type styling gowns in the salon for all chemical processes such as colouring, lightening and perming and more often than not, will wear them for cutting and styling too. However, a sleeveless cutting square is perfectly acceptable for "cutting only" services.

A clean, fresh towel is used to protect the client and their clothes from becoming wet during shampooing, or at any service provided at the basin. They also sit with a fastened towel around their shoulders when they are waiting to be attended to by the stylists at the styling units; after shampooing or when having a treatment. In addition to towels, salons provide plastic capes that can be worn over the top of towels to protect them and the clients from chemical spills or staining.

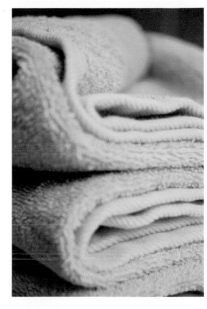

Clean, fresh towels are essential PPE for clients

Remember

Hazards	Check for
Floors	✔ Are they slippery or wet?
Doorways	✔ Are they clear of obstacles?
Electrical flexes	✔ Are they loose or trailing?
Chemicals	✔ Are they labelled and stored correctly?
Equipment	✔ Is it worn or in need of attention?

Activity

For this activity fill in the missing information in the table below.

Type of PPE	When is it used?	Why is it used?
disposable non-latex gloves		
gowns and towels		
stylist's waterproof apron		
barrier cream		
cotton wool		

Slips and trips

The most common cause of injuries at work is the "slip or trip". Resulting falls can be serious and a busy salon means lots of people – and the more clients there are, the more hair clippings there will be. Loose clippings left on the salon floor present a hazard to staff and clients alike. Both wet and dry hair clippings are easily slipped on, so make sure that you sweep the working areas regularly, and don't wait for stylists to finish; get

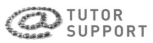

TUTOR SUPPORT

Activity 1.2 Matching: Identify hazards and evaluate the risks in your workplace Health and Safety at Work Act 1974

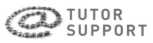

TUTOR SUPPORT

Activity 1.4 Reduce the risks to health and safety in your workplace chart

TUTOR SUPPORT

Activity 1.3 Task: Identify hazards and evaluate the risks in your workplace

rid of clippings before they build up. Clear them away from areas where people are working or walking and then brush them into a dustpan and put them into the waste bin. Wet floors are also a hazard within the salon, particularly in busy traffic thoroughfares. Any spillages must be cleared up immediately.

Look out for trailing leads. Portable electrical items such as blow dryers, tongs and straighteners plugged in at the styling unit can be a hazard to everyone, as it is very easy to trip on the lead.

Spillage and breakages

You do need to act quickly, but stop and think before doing anything.

1 First of all, what has been spilled or dropped?
2 Do you know what it is?
3 Is this something that needs special care and attention when handling?
4 Should you report the situation to someone else, or can you handle the situation yourself?
5 If you can, should you be wearing gloves?

Remember

If you are not sure about something, ask someone in authority.

Activity

What would you do if you found the following hazards?

Hazard	Sort it out myself		Report it	
Unsafe stacking of boxes in the stock room	Yes	No	Yes	No
Faulty kettle in the kitchen	Yes	No	Yes	No
Failed light bulb in the corridor	Yes	No	Yes	No
Spillage on the salon floor	Yes	No	Yes	No
A broken glass in the kitchen	Yes	No	Yes	No
Smoke appearing around the door of a closed room	Yes	No	Yes	No
Bare cable showing on the flex of a hand dryer	Yes	No	Yes	No

Supervisor's signature: . . . .   Date: . . . .

Preventing infection

Avoiding cross-infestation and cross-infection   Infection and disease occurs by two obvious methods within the salon/barber shop environment. It is either:

● brought in by a "carrier" visiting the salon who then cross-infects other people within the salon, or
● it is the result of poor hygiene and cleanliness within the salon.

A warm, humid salon can offer a perfect home for disease-carrying bacteria. If they can find food in the form of dust and dirt, they may reproduce rapidly. Good ventilation, however, provides a circulating air current that will help to prevent their growth. This is why it is important to keep the salon clean, dry and well aired at all times. This includes clothing, work areas, tools and all equipment.

Head lice and nits   This extremely common infestation can be very difficult to stop, particularly among young school children. Head lice are minute animal parasites that feed on the victim's blood. The infection can be observed in either the egg stage or the "adult" head louse stage, depending on how long the client has been infected. Head lice are passed from person to person through direct contact, and infestation is always accompanied by itching (caused by the parasite biting the scalp to feed on the host's blood). The adult louse lays eggs (called nits) and "cements" these to individual hairs close to the scalp. The incubation period is short and within days an immature louse emerges.

A number of products to combat head lice can be obtained from the chemist or, alternatively, from natural remedy sources and herbalists. Getting rid of the animal parasite is fairly easy, but it is much more difficult to destroy the nit. After an infected person has been treated with the shampoo or lotion, the nits need to be removed to break the head louse life cycle. The easiest way to remove the nits is to use a fine-tooth nit-comb when the hair is still wet. Applying vinegar (a mild acid solution) to the hair tightens the hair cuticle layer and makes it easier to comb away the nits. A final shampoo will remove any unpleasant smell and the hair is free from infestation.

Sterilisation   Sterilisation provides the most effective way of providing hygienically safe work implements in salons. Sterilisation means the complete eradication of living organisms. Different types of equipment use different sterilisation methods, which may be based on the use of heat, radiation or chemicals.

Ultraviolet radiation   Ultraviolet (UV) radiation cabinets can be used for storage of previously sterilised items, but they do not actually sterilise the items themselves.

Chemical sterilisation   Chemical sterilisers should be handled only with suitable personal protective equipment, as many of the solutions used are hazardous to health and should not come into contact with the skin. The most effective form of salon sterilisation is achieved by the total immersion of the contaminated implements into a jar of fluid.

Autoclave   The autoclave provides a very efficient way of sterilising using heat. It is particularly good for metal tools, although the high temperatures are not suitable for plastics such as brushes and combs. Items placed in the autoclave take around 20 minutes to sterilise. (Check with manufacturers' instructions for variations.)

See Chapter 4, GH3 Prepare for hair services and maintain work areas, for more information.

Working with electricity

Electricity can kill. Although deaths from electric shocks are very rare in hairdressing salons, even a non-fatal shock can cause severe and permanent injury. An electric shock from faulty or damaged electrical equipment may lead to a fall, for example, down a stairwell. Those using electricity may not be the only ones at risk. Poor electrical installations and faulty electrical appliances can lead to fires, which can also result in death or injury to others. Get into the habit of looking for loose cables and plugs on tongs, straighteners and hand dryers before plugging them in for use. If you think that a

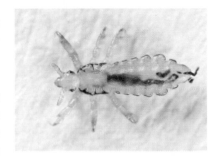
Microscopic image of a head louse

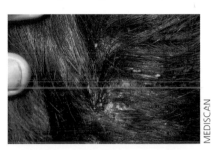
Nits cemented to individual hairs close to the scalp

MEDISCAN

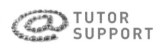
TUTOR SUPPORT

Task 1.4 Methods of sterilisation chart

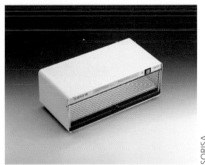
A UV radiation sterilizing cabinet

SORISA

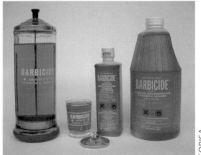
Barbicide™ – a common chemical disinfectant in the salon

SORISA

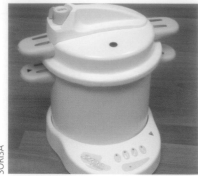

SORISA

The autoclave sterilises using heat

piece of electrical equipment is faulty or damaged, tell your supervisor immediately and they will label it making sure that no-one else tries to use it. For more information, see Electricity at Work Regulations 1989 in Appendix 1.

General salon hygiene

See Chapter 4, GH3 Prepare for hair services and maintain work areas.

Risks to health and safety

Emergencies   Other parts of this chapter have identified the health and safety situations where you need to contact specific members of staff about the issues affecting you in your work. That is not the only time when you need to alert others; there are situations where everyone needs to be informed. In emergencies such as fire, everyone must be alerted to the situation so that the building can be evacuated and people can make their way to the designated assembly point(s).

Activity

Find out where the fire extinguishers are kept on each floor of the premises. Write your answers in your portfolio.

1   What types of fire extinguisher are available in your premises?

2   What classes of fire are they meant to combat?

3   What is a fire blanket for?

4   What is your workplace policy for emergency evacuation?

5   Where are the alarms located?

6   Where are the emergency exits located?

Fire   All places of work must have adequate fire fighting equipment and means of escape. All fire exits have to be clearly marked with the appropriate signs and it must be possible to open all doors easily and immediately from the inside. The most likely reasons for fire occurring in a hairdressing salon are from:

● electrical faults – faulty wiring, overloading power sockets with multi-way adapters

● badly maintained equipment within the salon or staff only areas

● gas appliances left unattended

● badly positioned portable heaters – bottle gas space heaters, electric convector or fan heaters.

It is important to learn the evacuation process and practise it regularly. You need to know where the exits from the building are and where you need to regroup outside the building.

General evacuation rules   If a fire breaks out in the salon, the first thing that should be done is to raise the alarm. The person who discovers the fire should immediately tell the person in charge, who will then organise the evacuation. Staff should take responsibility for assisting clients to evacuate safely. No-one should stop to collect anything. Staff and clients should assemble at the assembly point and a senior member of staff should check that everyone is accounted for.

While this is being carried out a designated member of staff will call the fire brigade by dialling 999. If you have to do this then you will need to make sure that you have the right information ready to give the operator. You should never try and fight the fire yourself unless you have been properly trained to use the equipment and it is safe to do so. If it is safe to do so, all windows and doors should be closed as this will slow down the progress of the fire.

Fire fighting equipment

Fire fighting equipment must be available and located in specific areas. The equipment should only be used by properly trained people and only when it is safe to do so. It is very important that the right equipment is used. Using the wrong equipment could make the fire worse and endanger the person using it.

Different types of fire extinguishers are used to fight different types of fire and they are colour coded according to type. You must recognise types of fire extinguisher and be able to classify the type of fire in order to select the right type of fire fighting equipment. There are four classes of fire:

- **Class A**: Fires that involve solids such as paper, wood or hair.
- **Class B**: Fires that involve flammable liquids such as petrol.
- **Class C**. Fires that involve gases such as propane or butane.
- **Class D**: Fires that involve metals (not normally encountered in the salon).

All fire extinguishers are coloured red but have different coloured labels to show what the contents are. Fire extinguishers will be filled with one of four materials:

- **Water**: Colour code RED. These extinguishers are colour coded red and should only be used on **Class A** fires. They must not be used on fires involving electrical equipment.
- **Foam**: Colour code YELLOW. These extinguishers are colour coded yellow and are used on **Class B** fires and small Class A fires. They must not be used on fires involving electrical equipment.
- **Carbon dioxide**: Colour coded BLACK. These extinguishers are colour coded black and are used on **Class C** fires involving flammable gasses and burning liquids.
- **Dry powder**: Colour coded BLUE. These extinguishers are colour coded blue and are used on electrical fires.

There is also an extinguisher that contains a substance called BCF coloured Green. For **Class D** fires these would not normally be used in a salon environment.

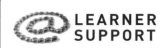
LEARNER SUPPORT
Health and safety puzzle

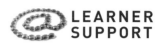
LEARNER SUPPORT
Health and safety quiz

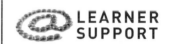
LEARNER SUPPORT
Health and safety wordsearch

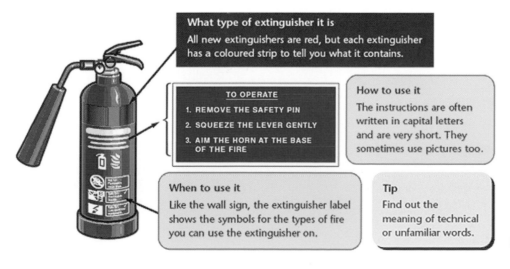

What type of extinguisher it is
All new extinguishers are red, but each extinguisher has a coloured strip to tell you what it contains.

TO OPERATE
1. REMOVE THE SAFETY PIN
2. SQUEEZE THE LEVER GENTLY
3. AIM THE HORN AT THE BASE OF THE FIRE

How to use it
The instructions are often written in capital letters and are very short. They sometimes use pictures too.

When to use it
Like the wall sign, the extinguisher label shows the symbols for the types of fire you can use the extinguisher on.

Tip
Find out the meaning of technical or unfamiliar words.

Diagram of a fire extinguisher

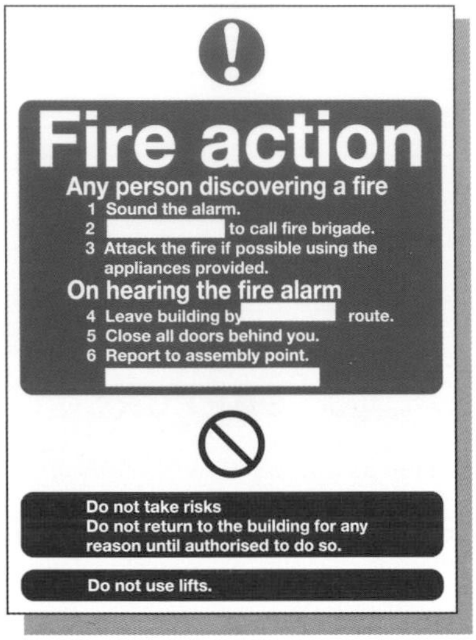

Fire action poster

TUTOR SUPPORT

Task 1.6 List: Reporting of diseases and dangerous occurrences regulations

EKU statement

G20 (eku11) where and when to get additional health and safety assistance

Accidents

Accidents will occur in the salon from time to time. In most cases these will be quite minor; sometimes they will be more serious. All accidents must be recorded in an **accident book** that must be kept in the salon. It should contain all the details of the accident, who was involved, how it happened, what action was taken, details of any witnesses, etc. If the accident is really serious then it must be reported to the Health and Safety Executive under the **Reporting of Injuries Diseases and Dangerous Occurrences Regulations** (RIDDOR). See Appendix 1 for more information. Accidents can be caused by any of the following:

- carelessness
- inappropriate behaviour
- tiredness
- misuse of substances (drink or drugs)
- faulty equipment
- poorly stored chemicals
- untidy and dirty work area
- poor salon layout.

The salon must have a first aid box that is properly stocked with all the necessary items needed to deal with minor accidents. The regulations also cover the need to provide qualified first aiders.

EKU *statement*

G20 (eku15) the importance of personal presentation in maintaining health and safety in your workplace

Dressing and behaving professionally

Personal appearance

The effort we put into getting ready for work reflects our pride in our work and that we care about what we do. Sometimes we have to wear things that we would not wear if we had a personal choice but professional standards and salon image must come first.

Remember

First impressions are lasting impressions: You don't get a second chance to create a good first impression.

Clothes   What we wear to work will be stated and con-firmed by the management of the salon. But whatever style and fashion we wear it should be practical and serviceable. Clothes should be easy to clean and iron if necessary and made of suitable fabrics. They should not be tight and restrictive, which would make working harder and more tir-ing; they may also make you perspire and increase **body odour (BO)**.

Shoes   Hairdressers and barbers should wear flat or low-heeled shoes that enclose the feet (cover the toes). We spend most of our time on our feet so comfortable shoes will help prevent backache.

Hair   As hair professionals, our hair is an advertisement of our skill in the salon. If your hair is a mess, think about how that affects our clients' confidence in you. Your hair should always look good and well styled to reflect the salon image. Your hair should always be clean, tidy and representative of the place where you work.

Make-up   If you wear make-up to work make sure that you check with your salon supervisor to see what is acceptable and appropriate.

Nails   You should have similar length, short, neatly mani-cured nails. Polish can be worn but must not be chipped or badly applied.

Jewellery   Wear only a minimum of jewellery while you are working. It can harbour germs, and it can be uncomfortable for the client because it can get tangled in the hair or injure the skin.

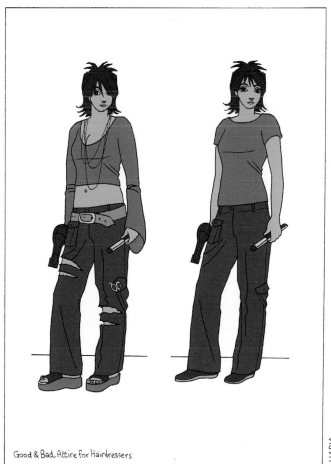

Good & Bad Attire for Hairdressers

© HABIA

The importance of personal appearance

Personal health, hygiene and behaviour

Hands and nails Make sure your hands are very clean. Dirty hands are not only unattractive, but also spread germs could and cross-infect your clients. Your hands are very important; they are the way you earn a living, so they need to be carefully looked after. Keep your nails clean, especially underneath, and try to keep them neatly mani-cured and not too long. Check them regularly for any disorders.

Always wash your hands before work, after using the toilet and after coughing or sneezing. This will reduce the risk of spreading infections to others. Use moisturising creams regularly to help replace the moisture lost by constant washing. When you shampoo, for example, it may be helpful to apply a moisturising cream. If the skin on your hands is allowed to become dry, it will crack and become very sore. This may prevent you from working until it heals.

Some people may suffer from dermatitis from exposure to all the chemicals used in the profession; if your hands continue to be sore and don't heal, consult your doctor. In some cases a person's sensitivity could mean that they have to give up their job.

Body The body has sweat glands all over its surface that are used to help control our body temperature by secreting moisture out on to the surface of the skin when you are hot. This provides a good breeding ground for bacteria, which in turn causes body odour (BO). It is essential that you have a shower or bath at least every day and use deo-dorants, anti-perspirants or similar.

Mouth Unpleasant breath (**halitosis**) can be offensive to others. It can be caused by all sorts of things: from things we have eaten, like onions or garlic, which are usually temporary; by smoking; stomach upsets; or other problems, such as pieces of food that get stuck between the teeth and then decay. As you will be working very close to the client, you will be breathing very close to them and so they will be able to smell any bad breath easily.

Remember

 In some salons and barber's shops you will find that a professional "uniform" will be the appropriate, permitted dress code. Other salons and shops have a dress code but on a less formal basis. You will know what is required and acceptable at your place of work from what is stated in your induction. Regardless of dress code you will always need to turn up for work in clean, ironed clothing.

EKU *statement*

G20 (eku16) the importance of personal behaviour in maintaining the health and safety of you and others

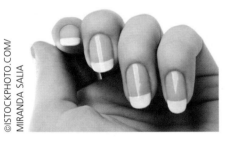

Similar length, short, neatly manicured nails

Remember

 Bad breath can easily be offensive to other people. To prevent bad breath brush your teeth regularly, particularly after eating, have regular dental checks and use a mouthwash or breath freshener. Dental type chewing gums work very well but may not be appropriate in the salon; always check with your salon supervisor first.

Remember

 If you use chemicals such as permanent wave lotion or colouring products, always wear disposable gloves. Not only does this protect your skin from chemical hazards, it will also stop your hands from being stained, which looks unprofessional.

Feet Like our hands, our feet are important because we do most of our work standing. We have looked at the sort of shoes we wear and must make sure they fit properly. You should also wash your feet regularly – some people's feet sweat a lot and this can cause foot odour. Make sure minor problems like veruccas, corns and athlete's foot are treated. Some disorders of the feet can make standing painful so you need to get them treated as soon as possible. Keep your toenails short: they should be cut/filed regularly so that they don't become painful during long periods of standing during the day.

Personal wellbeing   To work successfully as a hairdresser or a barber, you will need energy and stamina. Having a good health routine will give you that energy and stamina. The first aspect of that routine would be a well-balanced diet, one that is healthy and nutritious. You should take regular exercise; perhaps try playing sport or dancing. You should also get sufficient sleep and relaxation to help you recover from the stresses of the working day (it is often recommended that we have 8 hours of sleep a day).

Good posture is a must: as hair professionals we have to stand for long periods of time. Correct posture by standing properly will help prevent backache, and, in the long term, back problems and other conditions like varicose veins. Always stand with the back straight, your feet apart and your weight evenly distributed on both legs. Do not stand with all your weight on one of your legs and your pelvis tilted. If you stand like this for long periods you will get backache and possibly more serious problems with your lower back; you will also increase the risk of developing varicose veins.

The care and attention you pay to how you present ourselves for work is very important to your success and progress. Whatever job you do, make sure you look the part. Being thorough about our personal hygiene will ensure that you don't cause offence to anyone else, either to our clients or our colleagues. It can be embarrassing to be told you have a hygiene problem; the best way to avoid this is to make sure you don't have to be told.

Personal behaviour   The salon or barber's shop is a professional environment and you are on show. The way that you react to others and the respect that you show will be apparent not only by **what** you say, but **how** you say it. Treat others with a mutual, professional respect – regardless of what you think or would like to say.

Always conduct your work in a safe, professional manner; never fool around, as this could put others at risk by your actions or negligence. See Chapter 2, Unit G3 Contribute to the development of effective working relationships, for more information.

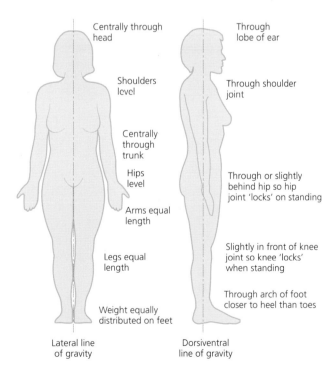

Correct standing posture

Labels (front figure): Centrally through head; Shoulders level; Centrally through trunk; Hips level; Arms equal length; Legs equal length; Weight equally distributed on feet; Lateral line of gravity

Labels (side figure): Through lobe of ear; Through shoulder joint; Through or slightly behind hip so hip joint 'locks' on standing; Slightly in front of knee joint so knee 'locks' when standing; Through arch of foot closer to heel than toes; Dorsiventral line of gravity

Remember

Always check your appearance before you start work, and don't forget to recheck throughout the day.

Remember

Coping with the stresses of hairdressing and barbering, which at times can be serious, is another thing we must learn to do.

Remember

Having a good diet and enough sleep as part of a good health routine will make sure that you can always give your best to the clients, your colleagues and your employer.

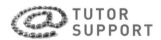
TUTOR SUPPORT

Task 1.7 Discuss personal hygiene

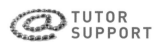
TUTOR SUPPORT

Task 1.8 Discuss good personal behaviour

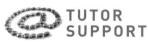
TUTOR SUPPORT

Activity 1.6 Health and safety wordsearch

Working in an environmentally friendly way

See Disposal of waste, page 58.

Checkerboard

I understand my job position and the impact of health and safety responsibilities associated with it ☐	I know who is responsible for health and safety and to whom to report any hazards in the workplace ☐	I always follow the salon's policy in respect to health and safety practices and procedures ☐

I can recognise the hazards and potential risks at work, and take appropriate action ☐

I know the main areas of potential risk for health and safety at work ☐

I understand all of the relevant health and safety regulations applicable to work ☐

I know why it is important to be aware of potential risks to personal health and safety ☐

I understand the implications of poor salon hygiene and cross-infection ☐

I can handle, use and work with materials, products and equipment safely ☐

I understand the necessity of personal hygiene and presentation ☐

I know the salon's policy and procedures in the event of fire or accidents ☐

I know what would be considered to be unsafe practices at work ☐

Revision questions

Q1 Fill in the blank: A hazard is something with a potential to cause _____.

Q2 Risk is the likelihood of the hazards potential being realised. True or false?

Q3 Which of the following are examples of hazards in the workplace? (You may choose more than one answer.)
1 hair clippings on the floor
2 plugged in appliances
3 trailing flexes across thoroughfares
4 products on retail shelves
5 difficult clients
6 blocked fire doors

Q4 If a comb is dropped on the floor during use it should be sterilised before it is used again. True or false?

Q5 Which of the following is considered to be an occupational health hazard? (Choose one answer.)
A head lice
B nits
C split ends
D dermatitis

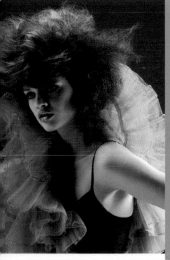

HAIR: NHF INSPIRE

Chapter**two**
Contribute to the development of effective working relationships

G3

G3.1

G3.2

G3.3

**CREDIT VALUE
FOR UNIT G3**
4 Credits

hit title

3 Contribute to the devel-
ment of effective working
ationships

is is a **mandatory** unit for
vel 1. It is made up
3 main outcomes.

ain outcomes

3 **(eku1)** Develop effective
rking relationships
h clients

3 **(eku2)** Develop effective
rking relationships with
lleagues

3 **(eku3)** Develop yourself
hin the job role

Unit G3: quick overview

What do I need to do for G3.1?

When **clients** are in the salon/barber's shop you need to:

- do things in a way that gives people confidence in your abilities
- put clients' belongings away carefully
- provide help to others without having to wait to be asked
- help clients if they need anything
- dress and behave professionally

What do I need to do for G3.2?

When working with other **staff members**, you need to:

- be friendly, helpful and respectful
- ask politely when you need help
- help willingly and promptly when asked
- only do jobs that you have been trained to do
- tell your supervisor about any problems

What do I need to do for G3.3?

You need to **improve yourself** within your job by:

- being able to gauge your own abilities
- asking other staff when you aren't sure
- learning new things
- reviewing your progress

Keywords

Appraisal

a process of reviewing work performance over a period of time

Body language

non-verbal communication provided by gestures, expressions and mannerisms

Goodwill

a way of treating clients in a kind, friendly and polite way that maintains their regular custom and favour

NVQ

an abbreviation for National Vocational Qualification: job-ready qualifications at a range of different levels

Personal development plan

an ongoing action plan for self improvement that defines personal objectives or targets, set over a period of time (often reviewed during appraisal)

EKU *statement*

G3 (eku7) how to communicate in a clear, polite, confident way and why this is important

G3 (eku8) the questioning and listening skills you need in order to find out information

G3 (eku6) your salon's guidelines for client care and why they should be followed

What things do I need to cover?

You need to **take part**:

- in training activities
- in salon services and operations
- by watching how others do their work

What things do I need to know?

You need to **know and understand**:

- what your job role covers
- when you need help or permission to do things
- why you must look, work, and act in the way that the salon manager expects
- how to communicate professionally and confidently with clients
- how to recognise when a client is angry or confused
- the standards of work expected by the manager
- why it is important to continue with your self improvement and personal development plan
- who you should ask for help when you are training
- how your NVQ relates to the things that you do at work

Introduction

You can see from the quick overview above that this chapter covers things that relate to the:

- salon's/barber's shop customers, who are referred to as **clients**
- other members of staff that you will be working with
- things that you need to do to improve yourself within your job role
- things that you can learn by taking part in different activities
- things that you need to know in order to do your job well.

Your ability to demonstrate professionalism will be put to the test

All of these things form the basis of what is called **professionalism**, and your ability to demonstrate professionalism in the salon will be put to the test. Having a good working relationship with both the clients and staff is an essential part of a successful business and you are very much part of that successful formula. Your contribution as a valued team member is like the last vital piece that finishes off the "jigsaw puzzle".

G3.1 Develop effective working relationships with clients

Do things in a way that gives people confidence in your abilities

Clients are the most important people in the salon; without them, there wouldn't be a salon to work in. As hairdressers, our approach to service is **customer focused** – putting the clients and their goodwill first, even if it means putting ourselves last. We want clients to enjoy themselves in the salon and to come back on a regular basis. The way you communicate can help.

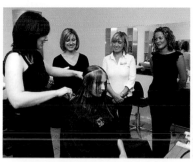

SAKS HAIR AND BEAUTY, WWW.SAKS.CO.UK

It is important that clients and hairdressers interact happily

The signs of good communication

The signs of good communication are:

- listening and responding to the clients' requests
- treating people with respect
- being confident, polite and courteous
- maintaining positive body language
- asking clients if they need anything.

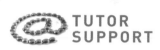

TUTOR SUPPORT

Discussion 2.1: Client relationships

Listening and responding to the clients' requests Show that you are listening by acting upon the information that clients give you. Let them finish what they are saying before you respond and never try to guess what they want or need: you may feel foolish if you get it wrong.

Treating people with respect Always treat clients with respect. People want and deserve to feel valued and you can do this by treating them in the same way that you would wish to be treated yourself. Try putting yourself in other people's situations and see things from their point of view. This is a special skill called **empathy**, and not everyone possesses this ability.

Being confident, polite and courteous Communicate clearly and confidently with clients at all times and you will make yourself understood too. The clients won't bite; they are genuinely interested in you and your contribution to the overall salon team. They will be impressed by your ability to talk confidently and comfortably about things that interest you. Try to remember that although confidence is important, being polite and courteous shows that you are interested in their wellbeing too. Always speak in a friendly way to clients and all those that you work with.

Maintaining positive body language Non-verbal communication is commonly referred to as **body language**. This is the unspoken way of letting others know what you really mean and think! When speaking to clients, try to maintain eye-to-eye contact; this infers that you are paying attention.

Always smile while you are speaking. This puts the client at ease and makes them feel welcome. This is particularly helpful and comforting to them as they may be feeling shy, timid or unsure themselves; it may even be their first visit to the salon and everything may be feeling very new or alien to them.

Remember

 Give clients the time to tell you what they want. Don't try to double guess them or try to anticipate their needs. You may be considered uncaring or rude.

Remember

 Beware: the messages that we provide through body language may be totally different to what we are saying as it may be SHOUTING just the opposite!

Remember

We express ourselves with body language through posture and gestures.
Here is a list of the most common:

1   Slouching looks unprofessional.
2   Folded or crossed arms portrays a closed mind or shows defensiveness.
3   Open palms indicates openness or honesty.
4   Scratching behind the ear or the back of the neck indicates uncertainty. Rubbing the nose whilst listening can indicate disbelief.
5   Inspecting fingernails or looking at a watch indicates boredom or vanity.
6   Talking with your hand in front your mouth may make the listener think you are dishonest.
7   Shifting from foot to foot shows that you're worrying about getting found out!

EKU *statement*

G3 (eku10) how to recognise when a client is angry and when a client is confused

Activity
What is the client saying?
Gestures and posturing are not the only ways that we show how we are feeling. Facial expressions show a lot about what we are thinking too.
Complete the missing information in the table below to indicate what each facial expression means and then answer the questions at the end.

Facial expression	What does it mean or show?
smiling	
frowning	
laughing	
narrowing of the eyes	
red cheeks and tight lips	

What sorts of facial expressions would a client be making if they were confused? Angry?

Remember

Time always passes more quickly for a client when there is something to read or look at.

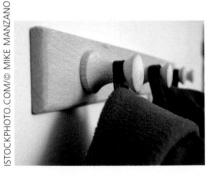

Ensure the client's belongings are safe and secure

Asking clients if they need things   Extend your politeness and courtesy by finding out when clients need things. Always make a point of asking if they would like a drink or something to read whilst they are waiting. This shows that they haven't been forgotten, even if their stylist is running a little late. Your courtesy and concern shows that you care and have noticed them and their needs.

Put clients' belongings away carefully

The receptionist's job is to manage the reception area, to attend to calls and receive the clients. It is a busy area and there is always something going on. Your job role extends to assisting them in what they are doing and you can show this by helping with clients.

When clients arrive at the salon, they will usually be carrying bags or be wearing a coat or jacket. If these items are not kept tidy and put away safely, they could become a **hazard** to other people or could get damaged.

For safety and security reasons, when a client arrives at the reception, take their belongings and put them away safely. Bags or shopping should be placed on the floor and not stored on pegs or on shelves as they might fall on someone, or damage the contents. Coats or jackets should be hung up on clothes hooks or placed upon coat hangers so that they don't lose their tailoring and become misshapen. Hang clients' coats or jackets away from the salon's styling gowns as these could easily be damp or stained with colour.

Provide help to others without having to wait to be asked

If a client needs help or advice, you should respond promptly and attend to their needs. Sometimes it will be something that you can do, such as turning the heat down on a dryer that is too warm or replacing a damp towel from around their shoulders with a clean, dry one. It could be getting magazines or simply something to drink. Whatever their request is, it is your duty to respond to their needs, but it doesn't necessarily mean that you can always sort out their problem yourself.

There will be occasions when you need to tell, or ask someone else if you are not able to help or you don't know the answer to what you are being asked. You will always be able to turn to a member of staff who does.

About things that you don't know

One of the most important rules for doing anything is "if you don't know the answer to a question, ask someone who does". This couldn't be more critical than in a work situation as all sorts of things could go wrong. So rather than worry about things that could go wrong, or for being responsible for things within the salon that are going wrong, you must put the accent on the positive. Therefore you **must** always ask others about things that you don't know. It is not a failing or weakness to ask others how things work, or what you need to do; on the contrary, it is a personal strength, as it shows that you really take an interest in your work and want to get things right.

Help clients if they need anything

Show that you are willing to provide a good service and gain the clients' trust in your abilities. Make sure that you always ask clients if they are comfortable and if they need anything. Good service never goes unnoticed. Whether it's the client, the other staff or your supervisor, people notice when people are making an effort – and when clients notice, they are more likely to express their gratitude and leave you a tip.

Dress and behave professionally

So far this chapter has looked at your professionalism in the way that you interact and relate to the clients by covering the aspects of spoken and unspoken communication. But there is another way that people make judgements about other people's abilities and professionalism.

When we meet someone for the first time, it is human nature to automatically create a first impression of what we see. This judgement, rightly or wrongly, is a lasting

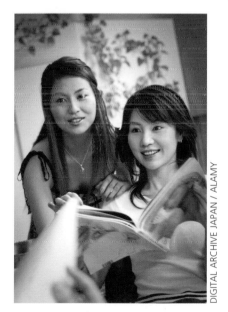

DIGITAL ARCHIVE JAPAN / ALAMY

Bringing clients magazines and drinks is an easy task that means a lot

Activity

The table below lists a number of situations that could occur within the salon. Think about the things that could go wrong and then:

1 Tick the first column if you can handle this yourself.

2 Then write down in the next column what you should do.

3 If you can't sort the problem, who do you seek help from?

Things that could go wrong	Can you sort this out yourself?	What should you do?	Who do you need to tell?
a client tells you that the colour on her head is beginning to feel sore			
a client spills her coffee on the styling section shelf			
you see that a client's towel is wet and has fallen to the floor			
after a client has been finished, you find that they have left their purse on the side			
a client has had a perm and is waiting for it to develop – but you notice that the lotion is dripping down around their face			
a stylist finishes a dry cut on a client and leaves the styling section untidy			

Remember

 If in doubt always ask another member of staff. There will be lots of things that you don't know, but that's what training is for – finding out and learning the things that you need to know in order to do your job correctly.

impression and in a professional environment it has to be the right one. Your professionalism is conveyed to the clients by:

- the way that you dress, in what you wear and how you wear it
- your appearance, i.e. your tidiness, cleanliness and your hair
- the way you behave and relate to other members of staff.

This is why different jobs have different dress codes. Your salon will have its own dress code and expected standards of behaviour and appearance and you must abide by these rules. These will be the minimum levels that management will accept.

Remember

 It is human nature to try to rationalise and assess everything we see. We do this when we meet new people in less than 10 seconds. You don't get a second chance to make a good first impression!

Activity

Find out what your salon's expected standards are in relation to:

1 what you should wear for work

2 how you should look, in respect to your hair, make up and general appearance

3 how you should behave when working

4 how you should respond to the clients.

Activity

Complete the activity by filling in the missing information in the table below to explore how different people in different jobs dress, then give reasons why.

Type of job	Dress code	Reason
a personal trainer in a fitness club		
a soldier on parade		
a chef cooking in a kitchen		
a beauty therapist		
a hair stylist or barber		
a check-out operator in a supermarket		

EKU *statement*

G3 (eku2) when you need to seek agreement with or permission from others

G3 (eku3) why it is important to work within your job responsibilities and what might happen if you do not do so

G3 (eku4) the standards of behaviour that are expected of you when working in the salon, including attendance and punctuality

G3 (eku5) your salon's standards for personal appearance

G3 (eku21) why good working relationships are important

G3 (eku24) who to report to when you have difficulties in working with others

G3.2 Develop effective working relationships with colleagues

Be friendly, helpful and respectful

All the staff in the salon work as a team, and your contribution is equally important. Without this joint effort, nothing will happen: the stylists, colourists and technicians won't be able to do their jobs and your fellow juniors won't be able to do theirs. Therefore it is essential that you are friendly, helpful and respectful to other staff at all times. You may have your differences away from the salon floor, but you are now in a professional working environment and any animosity (bad feelings) must be left behind.

The friendships that you make out of work are different and made out of choice, whereas those acquaintances made through work are based on team associations. The two relationships are very different and require margins for tolerance, patience and acceptance, which happen to be part of your professional development within the job role.

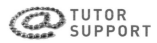

TUTOR SUPPORT

Discussion 2.2: Why are relationships with colleagues important?

Ask politely when you need help

The work carried out by staff within the salon depends on good communication, and that means politely asking others for help as well as offering help. Communication is a two-way process and it is always welcomed and returned. You ask for help or advice in a friendly manner and someone else responds to your needs with respect.

Remember

 Be courteous and considerate at all times; ask for help politely and you will always be treated with respect.

Help willingly and promptly when asked

Good team working promotes a happy salon, and in turn this creates an atmosphere that everyone will sense. On the other hand, a team that doesn't gel together creates a stilted or strained bad atmosphere that clients will notice. You can help to prevent this from happening by always being willing to provide your assistance. Your eagerness and promptness to take part or help won't go unnoticed and will pay you back in the longer term.

Activity

Look at the statements on the left and match them up with the corresponding statement on the right.

Relationships at work are based upon	personal preferences and choice
Friendships outside work are based upon	effective communication takes place
Customer care is built on	mutual respect and teamwork
Good customer relations occur when	professionalism and personal service
Teamwork takes place when	making the best of personal strengths and working to improve weaknesses
Self-development in the job role means	all the staff do their jobs efficiently

Know the hazard symbols

EKU *statement*

G3 (eku23) how to manage your time effectively

Only do jobs that you have been trained to do

Safety is always your employer's first consideration and a lot of things will have gone on behind the scenes to make the place that you work in fit for purpose. But that doesn't mean that work is always hazard free. Providing a public access to premises for a place of work always creates situations where accidents or hazards can occur, so you too play an important role in helping to prevent those hazards from occurring. One of the ways in which you can do this is to only do things that you have been shown to do. Put another way, never try to do any job that you haven't been trained to do, or you are unsure about – this may put the safety of yourself, or other people at risk.

Remember

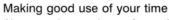 **Making good use of your time**

Always make good use of your time when you are in the salon because there are always things that needs doing. Sometimes you will have to juggle what you are doing as you may be asked to do one job whilst carrying out another for someone else:

- Keep a list of the different tasks you have been asked to do and that way you won't get into trouble for forgetting anything.
- Find out what jobs have priority – some things are more important or urgent. Do these things first.
- If you don't understand your task, ask someone to explain it right away.
- If you have to leave something halfway through, make sure that you complete it at the earliest convenient moment.

Tell your supervisor about any problems

Whenever you do encounter something new, or are unsure about doing something, tell either your supervisor or a senior member of staff, or ask for their assistance.

G3.3   Develop yourself within the job role

Being able to gauge your own abilities

Being able to self-assess your own skills at work is an important part of your on-going development and meeting your training targets. The key to doing your job and performing your team role properly is knowing what you do well and what you don't. On the face of it; some tasks seem very simple and other seem very hard. Why is that? Tasks that we do repeatedly become simpler. However, there are other jobs that we don't do so often or dislike. These are the ones where we feel "out of our comfort zone" and that uncertainty, or self doubt makes us feel that we can't do them properly. Assessing your own strengths and weaknesses requires you to be realistic and honest with yourself about your capabilities. You need to define those jobs that you know and do well and those that you don't. The list of things that you don't do well forms the basis for creating targets for your personal development plan.

EKU *statement*

G3 (eku15) how to identify your own strengths and weaknesses

G3 (eku16) the importance of continuous professional development

G3 (eku17) who can help you identify and obtain opportunities for your development and/or training

Activity
Strengths and weaknesses
This activity will help you to identify your own strengths and weaknesses.
Complete this activity by putting a tick in the appropriate boxes for each of the skills listed in the table. When you have filled in the information below ask your work supervisor to check your responses.

Personal Skill	I do this	I do this well	I don't do this	I don't do this very well
communicating with clients				
communicating with work colleagues				
helping other staff in their work				
doing things myself without having to be told all the time				
dealing with clients and handling their queries				
tidying the salon and keeping things clean				

Asking other staff when you aren't sure

You can find out how well you are getting on by getting feedback from the people that you work with. Ask the stylists if you are doing things properly. As you work with them on a day-to-day basis, they will be able to tell you how well you are doing. However, it's one thing

EKU statement

G3 (eku9) the rules and procedures regarding the methods of communication you use

G3 (eku18) how using the National Occupational Standards for Hairdressing can help you identify your development needs

G3 (eku19) how to access information on National Occupational Standards and qualifications, relevant to hairdressing

G3 (eku20) the importance of continually using and updating your own personal development plan

LEARNER SUPPORT

Contribute to effective working relationships wordsearch

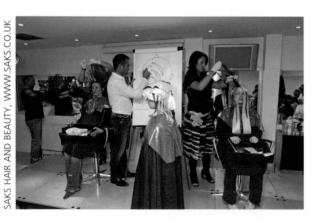

SAKS HAIR AND BEAUTY, WWW.SAKS.CO.UK

Learning through a formal training event at a salon

Remember

For more information about National Vocational Qualifications for hairdressing and beauty see www.habia.org.

asking the people that you get on well with about your abilities. Often, their comments will only cover the positives! Your friends are helpful and supportive, but they are not necessarily qualified, and probably don't want to hurt your feelings. Ultimately, your work supervisor will be the one who has a very clear idea of what you can do, where you are now and where you need to be. At work, this assessment of your skills is called **appraisal**.

> **Activity**
> Find out how you are expected to communicate with other staff and clients in your salon. Write the answer in your portfolio.

Learning new things

If you are "willing and open" to learn new things, then there are many ways to make this happen at work. The phrase "willing and open" is key: someone who **wants** to learn will always get more out of learning opportunities than someone who **doesn't**.

At school you had to attend classes covering a range of different subjects, some of which you may have enjoyed and/or found easy, whereas others you may not have enjoyed and/or found difficult. At the end of a learning period or syllabus, you then had to take exams or an assessment. The world of work is very different: you have to learn **everything** that is related to the job. Some of these things are fun and easy to learn, but others may be more difficult to follow or understand, or just plain boring! You will find that learning opportunities present themselves in all sorts of ways and you should make the most of these in order to get on well. Learning opportunities fall into two categories: the ones that rely upon your participation in through formal training events, and others that rely upon your ability to learn through informal, day-to-day routine activities.

Formal learning and training could take place during work hours or could be arranged as an evening, or outside-of-work event. Most salons have specific times for staff training, usually model evenings, role plays or demonstrations and presentations. For example, a junior stylist may demonstrate how a professional shampoo is carried out for you to practise afterwards. Alternatively, a manufacturer's field technician may do an in-salon product demonstration.

You will find that you learn most things informally through your everyday duties; you will be seeing how other staff do things, how staff communicate with clients and handle situations. You will hear how they offer services or recommend products and how they apply products when they are showing the clients how they are used. Informal learning opportunities crop up all the time and it is your responsibility to learn when you are working.

Reviewing your progress

Earlier in this chapter we use the term **appraisal**. The appraisal interview is not an inquisition, nor is it a "witch hunt" or a way of "having a go" at you. It is a positive and professional process, and your positive contribution is important. The appraisal process is a way of looking at an individual's abilities, assessing their needs and mutually agreeing a future course of action.

Activity

What can you learn here?

The table below lists a number of situations which are opportunities to learn. Think about what is happening in each situation and then complete the missing information. When you have finished check your answers with your work supervisor.

Learning opportunity	What can you learn from this?	What questions would you ask?
watching a junior carrying out a shampoo		
helping the receptionist		
helping the stylist by passing up		
watching the stylist mixing chemicals		
listening to a stylist conduct a consultation		
helping the junior refill the shampoos and conditioners		

A business needs to do well in order to survive and you are an essential part of that team. You will not know how you are doing unless someone in a supervisory role gives you feedback. The appraisal process provides this mechanism.

In order for the business to do well and keep everyone employed, it must create a profit. If a business does not make a profit then it soon ceases to exist! Therefore, the business must achieve its performance targets in order to survive and prevail. Likewise, you are part of that entity and you must achieve your personal targets so that the business can achieve its targets and your personal targets and objectives are set out within your appraisal. The appraisal interview provides a way of:

- reviewing the progress that has been made in work since the last appraisal
- checking and formalising current personal performances
- setting new targets; moving on, from what has already been learned and agreeing new, realistic targets that can be achieved by the next appraisal.

Many salons would expect a learner to achieve NVQ Level 1 within their first year and in most cases, the target of Level 1 will be a "milestone" on route to obtaining Level 2. So unless there was a system for giving people feedback on how well they are doing, how would they know where they are on their personal learning journey? Your review of progress will be done with your supervisor during your appraisal. This will give you the opportunity to see where you are now and where you need to be.

Where you are now

When you started work you were given a job description. In many ways it looks like a sort of checklist and that's because it covers all the things that you do in your work. Now, depending how long you have been in the role, you may be able to say that you have covered certain of the duties already. Some of these things will be done well and others, perhaps not so well. Your appraisal will be an opportunity to look at these things and discuss your progress and competence in each of the tasks associated with them. Then after discussing the things that you can do, you can talk about the things that you need to work on and do in the future. Be positive and willing to contribute; discuss the things that

EKU *statement*

G3 (eku1) your job role and responsibilities and how this relates to the role of other team members

G3 (eku11) how to get information about your job, your work responsibilities and the standards expected of you

G3 (eku13) your personal development targets and timescales

G3 (eku14) the importance of meeting your work targets

G3 (eku22) how to react positively to reviews and feedback and why this is important

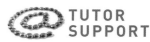

TUTOR SUPPORT

Discussion 2.3: Job description

TUTOR SUPPORT

Short answer tests

EKU statement

G3 (eku12) your salon's appeal and grievance procedures

you feel you do well and have completed. Be objective and not defensive as this is an aid to your personal development and not a personal attack.

Where you need to be

When the "where you are now" has been discussed and agreed, its time to think towards the future. Quite simply, you and your supervisor have looked at the targets that were set during the last appraisal; you have identified where these have been achieved, and then jointly, set out a mutually agreed plan for the future. These targets will be "tailored" to your abilities and pace of learning, but will clearly define in a plan of action: what you need to do in order to get to where you need to be.

Activity
Sample job description

Job description – Junior/Trainee

Location	Cutz 'n Curlz
Main purpose of job:	to provide good customer care at all times
	maintain a good standard of client care, follow salon's standard training practices and procedures

Candidate specification

The candidate should:

- have a professional level of interpersonal/communication skills
- be a willing and conscientious team member
- be willing to participate in personal development activities during work hours and on training evenings
- achieve designated performance targets
- undertake duties requested by senior staff

To maintain company policy in respect of:

- personal standards of health/hygiene
- personal standards of appearance/conduct
- operating safely whilst at work
- timekeeping and service provision
- company image and public promotion
- company security practices and procedures

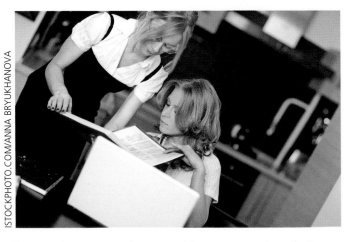

Always take up any grievance with your supervisor first

Your salon's appeal and grievance procedure

A grievance is a complaint or objection to something that has happened. It could occur for a number of reasons where you may feel that you have been treated unfairly or wrongly and in a work situation this could relate to many things. If you have a grievance at work, you must deal with the situation professionally. Be calm and sensible and take it up with your work supervisor first. If that would be a problem for you, seek independent advice on how to deal with the situation.

Sometimes disputes cannot be sorted out easily, and in these circumstances, a formal salon procedure comes into play.

Your salon will have its own way of implementing grievance or disciplinary procedures, and you should receive this information during your induction. The procedure will cover the following issues:

- conflict at work between staff
- unfair (or presumed unfair) treatment at work (e.g. being asked to do tasks beyond your abilities or unsafe practices)
- discrimination in any situation.

Remember

Your salon has a procedure for appeals and grievances. See the company's handbook or speak to your work supervisor or employer for more information.

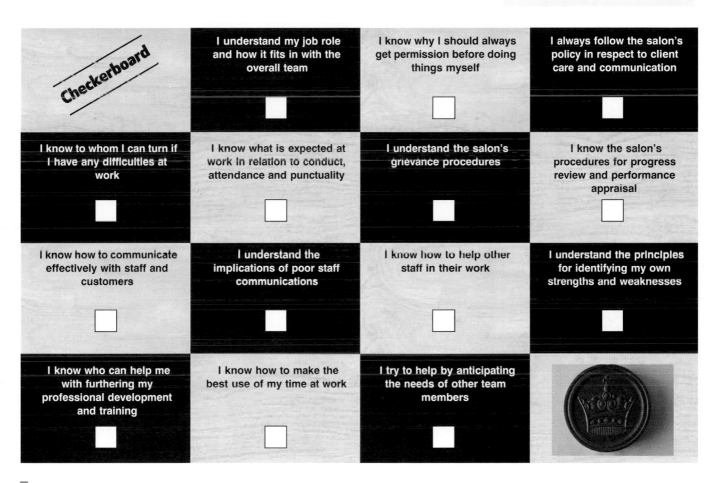

Checkerboard

| I understand my job role and how it fits in with the overall team ☐ | I know why I should always get permission before doing things myself ☐ | I always follow the salon's policy in respect to client care and communication ☐ |

| I know to whom I can turn if I have any difficulties at work ☐ | I know what is expected at work in relation to conduct, attendance and punctuality ☐ | I understand the salon's grievance procedures ☐ | I know the salon's procedures for progress review and performance appraisal ☐ |

| I know how to communicate effectively with staff and customers ☐ | I understand the implications of poor staff communications ☐ | I know how to help other staff in their work ☐ | I understand the principles for identifying my own strengths and weaknesses ☐ |

| I know who can help me with furthering my professional development and training ☐ | I know how to make the best use of my time at work ☐ | I try to help by anticipating the needs of other team members ☐ | |

Revision questions

Q1 Fill in the blank: The correct name for salon or barber shop customers is _____.

Q2 Relationships at work are different to those outside of work. True or false?

Q3 Which of the following are examples of good teamwork? (You may choose more than one answer.)

1 asking for help politely from others
2 preparing trolleys with curlers
3 sitting at the reception desk
4 finding ways to avoid jobs
5 finding ways to learn new things
6 cleaning the brushes for the stylists

Q4 Goodwill is shown by treating clients in a kind friendly way. True or false?

Q5 Which of the following would not be a feature of a self-development plan? (You may choose more than one answer.)

1 self improvement
2 setting targets
3 personal objectives
4 grievance procedures

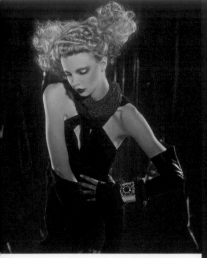

HAIR: RICHARD WARD, PHOTOGRAPHY: DANIELE CIPRIANI

Chapter**three**

Assist with salon reception duties

G2

G2.1

G2.2

G2.3

**CREDIT VALUE
FOR UNIT G2**

Unit title

G2 Assist with salon reception duties

This is an **optional** unit for Level 1. It is made up of 3 main outcomes.

Main outcomes

G2 (eku1) Maintain the reception area

G2 (eku2) Attend to clients and enquiries

G2 (eku3) Help to make appointments for salon services

Unit G2: quick overview

What do I need to do for G2.1?

You will be **maintaining the reception** area by:

- keeping all areas clean and tidy
- monitoring stationery and product levels
- looking out for faulty or damaged products
- demonstrating good customer care

What do I need to do for G2.2?

You will be **attending to clients and visitors** by:

- handling enquiries politely and positively
- informing the stylists that their clients have arrived
- referring enquiries you can't handle
- taking messages for others
- handling information in a confidential way

What do I need to do for G2.3?

You will be helping to **make appointments for clients** by:

- dealing with requests promptly and politely
- accurately recording appointments
- requesting assistance when needed
- confirming and recording details correctly

What things do I need to cover?

You will be **handling appointments and enquiries**:

- face to face when clients and people come into the salon

- on the telephone

What things do I need to know?

You need to **know and understand**:

- your salon's procedures for making accurate appointments

- the limits of your authority in reception

- the reasons for maintaining confidentiality

- who you refer to when you have problems

- how to take and deliver messages for others

- how to ask, answer and generally communicate with clients in a professional way

- the salon's services and treatments, their duration and pricing

- the salon's retail product range, it's pricing and how to spot faulty or damaged goods

- the stationery and systems used at reception

Keywords

Appointment system
the efficient way of organising salon work

Client care
maintaining goodwill whilst developing regular, repeated business

Confidentiality
the professional way of handling client information

Effective communication
professional communication that is not ambiguous, providing clear instruction or information

Introduction

The reception is the most important area of the salon, as it is here that the client makes their first contact with the business. It is here that appointments are made, clients pay for their services and people and visitors come and go. This chapter is about helping with salon reception duties.

The reception is the hub of any busy salon

You will have to show that you can keep the reception area neat and tidy, greet people entering the salon, deal with their questions and make straightforward appointments. You will be using your communication skills when people come into the salon, or when speaking to them on the telephone. This is a very important part of the business and you will be contributing to that overall team effort.

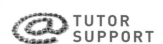

TUTOR SUPPORT

Task 3.4 Why reception duties are important

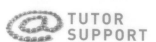

TUTOR SUPPORT

Task 3.1 Discuss - First impressions of the salon

EKU *statement*

G2 (eku2) the limits of your authority when maintaining the reception area

G2 (eku2) the limits of your authority when attending to people and enquiries

G2 (eku2) the limits of your authority when making appointments

G2 (eku8) the importance to the salon's business of effective communication

G2 (eku18) what and how much reception stationery should be kept at your reception area

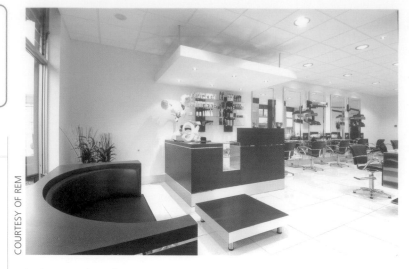

COURTESY OF REM

A clean, welcoming salon reception area

First impressions

The reception area is the first point of contact that the clients have with the salon and you may be the first person in the salon that they come into contact with. Their opinion will be influenced by that first impression, in what they see and the way in which they are handled. How you greet them and how you handle yourself is key to the success of everything that happens next.

G2.1   Maintain the reception area

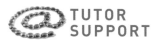

TUTOR SUPPORT

Task 3.2 List: Reception standards

Keeping all areas clean and tidy

Salon tidiness is essential and maintenance in reception is equally important: a clean, attractive reception and retail display conveys a message of professionalism and pride. Add to this a warm smile, a friendly "Hello, how can I help you?" and good eye contact and instant, good customer care takes place.

Remember

Put yourself in the client's position. What do they see? Are the product labels facing the front? Is there supporting product information available? Is everything clean? How would you feel if you picked up a product and it left a dirty, dusty ring on the shelves?

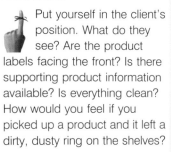

"Hello, how can I help you?"

Is your salon reception area clean and tidy? It is your duty to make sure that the area is clean and tidy at all times; make sure that carpets are vacuumed before the salon gets busy and that tiled areas are swept or mopped (and kept dry) throughout the day. Keep the displays fully stocked and the shelves free of dust. Check retail products for condition and ensure price labels are clearly visible. Attractive retail products will encourage clients to look at what is on offer and find out more. Is the salon's reception desk tidy? The **appointment system** is in continual use, so stationery, pens and messages can be left around. The desk is the focal point of any reception and how things are organised will affect how clients view the salon.

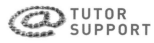

TUTOR SUPPORT

Task 3.3 Procedure:
Maintaining the reception area

Activity

Client communication

Watch how the people in the reception area deal with clients and enquiries. What do you notice about the way they do the following things?

Aspect of service	What happens next?
a client arrives at reception	
the telephone rings	
someone leaves a message for one of the stylists	
a client is browsing the products on the retail display	

Now write the answers to the following questions in your portfolio. What are you expected to do in respect to:

1 Maintaining the reception area?

2 Attending to people and enquiries?

3 Making appointments?

Monitoring stationery and product levels

The reception area is always busy with clients arriving or wanting to pay their bill; the telephone is often ringing with clients wanting to make appointments. Therefore the desk must be well organised. Stationery, such as memo pads, pens and till rolls or electronic payment machine stationery should be checked each morning before the salon opens and restocked throughout the day.

Don't forget the product information: promotional information helps to sell retail products. It provides them with relevant information in professionally produced leaflets, booklets and brochures. Make sure that all current promotions have their supporting information at hand.

In busy, thriving salons the contents of the retail displays are going to change throughout the day. The salon may start out with fully stocked displays, but as the items are sold, gaps will start appearing and product lines may run out. A well-stocked display is more appealing than one with gaps. If you notice any shortages, get some replacements out of the stock storage room.

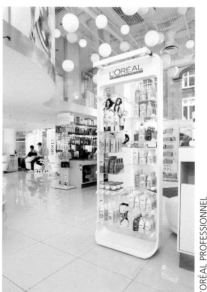

A well-stocked display will appeal to clients

L'ORÉAL PROFESSIONNEL

Checklist
Salon tidiness

✔	desk dusted and tidied before clients arrive
✔	appointment diary close to hand and ready for use

✔	card payment receipt rolls and till rolls replenished and spares available
✔	stationery stocks checked and replenished
✔	shelves and retail products dusted or wiped
✔	missing items or low stock levels replaced or reported
✔	damaged or faulty product packaging removed and reported to the manager
✔	products rearranged and gaps in product lines removed from displays
✔	product information and pricing is up to date, close at hand and easy to read
✔	product promotions are clearly displayed, public information is available and the correct product items are arranged appropriately according to the current offer or promotion

Remember

 Dust the products on the retail displays regularly: no-one wants to handle products that look murky and dull, regardless of how fabulous they are and what they can do.

 Activity

Positive and negative impressions

Complete the activity by putting yourself in the client's position and thinking about the following things. What things would give you a positive impression and what things would give you a negative impression of the business? Make a copy of the table to keep in your portfolio.

Aspect of salon/service	A positive impression	A negative impression
you open the door and walk into reception		
you walk over to look at the products		
a member of staff makes eye contact with you		
you want to make an appointment		
you feel confused about what you are hearing		
you ask to speak to the manager		

EKU *statement*

G2 (eku1) what to look for to identify any faults in products as they are being prepared for sale (e.g. damage, loose packaging, cracks, leaks, etc.)

Remember

 Show clients you cared for them by offering a drink whilst they are waiting. It shows that they are being attended to and haven't been forgotten. Remember to ask how they take it.

Looking out for faulty or damaged products

Sometimes accidents happen and a product's packaging can get damaged. If you find any products that are faulty or have been damaged, report them to the person in charge of the stock and then clear up any spillages or leaks. Look for faulty stock as you prepare it for display. Look out for leaked products in the delivery packaging. If any of the contents are missing a product cannot be sold. Retail products are often packed in sealed boxes in multiples of 6s, 10s or 12s, and each one has a cost to the salon. All damaged items can be legally returned to the supplier and the costs reimbursed, so by reporting them to your supervisor, you will be showing your efficiency and making savings for the salon.

Demonstrating good customer care

Remember that some salons provide a basic service and others a premium service. The contents of a service are defined by the business, but even the minimum service should always maintain a good level of hospitality.

Activity

Find out what your salon or shop provides as its general hospitality. What is the customer service policy at your salon? What aspects of the service are complimentary? Write your answers in your portfolio.

Some salons offer drinks as part of their service policy; make sure that you offer the client whatever your salon includes as part of its customer service policy. Always make a point of asking if they would like something to read. A style book is particularly helpful as it may save valuable time when the stylist does the client's consultation, or it might even get them thinking about something new. If they don't want to look at styles, perhaps get them a magazine instead.

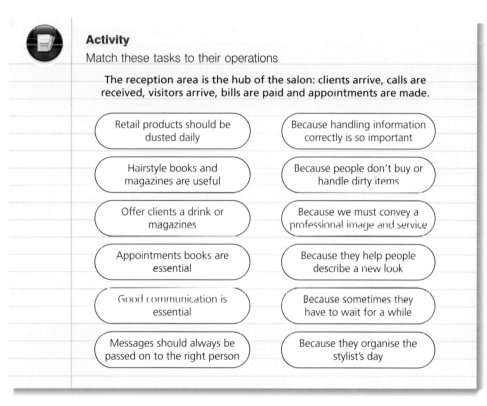

Activity

Match these tasks to their operations

The reception area is the hub of the salon: clients arrive, calls are received, visitors arrive, bills are paid and appointments are made.

Retail products should be dusted daily	Because handling information correctly is so important
Hairstyle books and magazines are useful	Because people don't buy or handle dirty items
Offer clients a drink or magazines	Because we must convey a professional image and service
Appointments books are essential	Because they help people describe a new look
Good communication is essential	Because sometimes they have to wait for a while
Messages should always be passed on to the right person	Because they organise the stylist's day

Remember

When you find magazines for the client, pick the latest. Old magazines are more suited to a dentist's or doctor's office than a fashion conscious salon!

EKU *statement*

G2 (eku1) your salon's procedures for client care at reception

G2 (eku4) who to refer to with different types of enquiries

G2 (eku9) how and when to ask questions

G2 (eku10) how to say things that suit the purpose of your discussion

G2 (eku11) how to speak clearly in a way that suits the situation

G2 (eku12) how to show you are listening closely to what people are saying to you

G2 (eku13) how to adapt what you say to suit different situations (ie the amount you say, your manner and tone of voice)

G2.2 Attend to clients and enquiries

Handling enquiries politely and positively

Effective communication is essential in a service industry like hairdressing or barbering and it is crucial to the businesses success at reception. The way that you address people that arrive at the salon is going to leave them with a lasting impression. Your communication needs to be clear and effective with everyone. Some people aren't as able as others, so sometimes you will have to speak a little more slowly or perhaps a little louder. In any situation, make sure that you have been understood by confirming the details back to them.

Communication is about passing information from one to another. The information a message can provide includes details, advice or answers. The content of the message

TUTOR SUPPORT

Task 3.6 Discuss/List: Positive impression

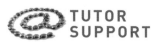

TUTOR SUPPORT

Task 3.5 Communication

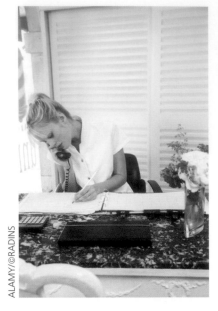

Good telephone communication depends on your voice alone

is reinforced by the way that it is said – by the extra information that you provide both consciously and subconsciously; in the tone of your voice and the expressions or gestures you make. Be polite and positive at all times: your ability to do your job will be assumed (rightly or wrongly) by the way in which you communicate with the clients. When you are speaking in a:

- strained voice: this indicates that "I'm under pressure here, don't bother me now"
- raised voice: this indicates that "I'm angry about what has just happened over there"
- friendly voice: this indicates that "I'm helpful, professional and I'm ready to serve".

Not everyone that arrives at the salon is a client, and unless you establish this first, you could embarrass yourself. You need to verify who you are dealing with and what they want. The simplest greeting for a face-to-face communication is to smile and say "How may I help you?". This polite and friendly greeting provides a "blanket" address for any visitor and allows them to respond with. "I have an appointment to see…" or "I would like to make an appointment…" or "Is Jill busy? I would like a quick word". Then, depending on their response, you can adapt your reply. Review the section on body language in Chapter 2, page 25, for more information about communication.

EKU statement

G2 (eku14) how to show positive body language

G2 (eku16) the products available for sale and their cost

Activity
Retail products in your place of work

Complete the missing information in the following table.

Retail product name	Who makes the product?	What is it used for?	How much does it cost?

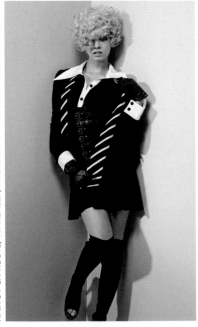

Informing the stylists that their clients have arrived

When the client arrives for their appointment, make sure that you attend to them promptly; confirm their appointment and the time and then direct them to a seat. Always make a point of making them feel welcome. People hate being made to wait, and this can start their experience off on the wrong foot. If you think of those times when you have to wait in a queue or wait to be seen by the doctor, those feelings and memories will spring to mind. In a salon or barber's shop this time **belongs** to the client, it should be treated as something that they **own**, and therefore it is not our right to take that away.

It is said that one of the greatest gifts that you can give is your time, and you can demonstrate this by being aware of other people's time. When a client arrives for an appointment, you must inform the stylist immediately. If a client has to wait because a stylist is running late, you can at least inform them so that they can look at their alternatives.

Remember

When making appointments, try to offer a range of dates at different times for the client. If a client can't make an appointment in the week around 3.30 pm she may be at work, so offering another day at the same time will probably be unsuitable too.

Referring enquiries you can't handle

Enquiries made either in person "face to face" or on the telephone should be handled in the same way. In both instances we need to respond promptly and politely. If you don't know the answer to a question, ask someone who does – accurate information is essential. So stop! Listen to what is being said, hear the request and react on the information or instruction. Misinterpreting what has been said could result in giving or recording the wrong information. Misinterpretation when making appointments can turn into a disaster – imagine if the client turns up on the wrong day and can't be done because her stylist is too busy!

It is even more difficult on the telephone because callers can only gain an impression of the salon from the person they are speaking to. This person becomes the salon's sole representative, acting on behalf of the business, and his or her ability to listen, speak clearly, respond to requests and act upon information is critical to the salon's **goodwill** and image.

Smile when you answer the telephone – people will "hear" the friendliness in your voice. Speak clearly so that the caller understands everything you say. After listening to the caller's request, confirm the main points back to the caller. This summarises the information and ensures that all details are correct. Keep the call short: calls cost money and waste valuable salon time.

There will be occasions when you need to seek the assistance or advice from others. Recognising situations when you are unable to help is not a failure – it is all part of professional communication. Some situations will require the attention of someone else; imagine when the window cleaner arrives and says "Shall I just get on with it" or requests payment, or when stock arrives and a signature is required for taking delivery and accepting the condition of the goods.

Taking messages for others

You will sometimes need to take a message on behalf of someone else. It is essential that these messages are accurately recorded and delivered promptly to the appropriate person. When taking messages, always make sure that you record the time and date, and make clear who the message is for and who it is from. Then give as much detail as you can in relation to the context of the message:

- who the message is for
- who has taken it
- the date and time received
- the purpose or content of the message.

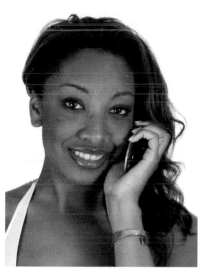

You are the salon's representative when speaking on the telephone

EKU *statement*

G2 (eku1) your salon's procedures for taking messages

G2 (eku7) the importance of taking messages and passing them on to the right person at the right time

Remember

Always keep a message pad close to the telephone: writing messages on the appointment book is unprofessional and must be avoided at all costs.

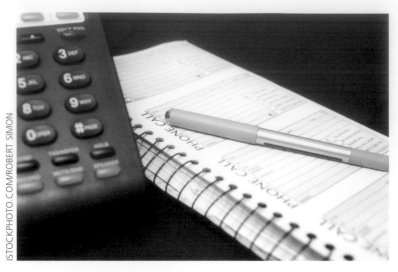

ISTOCKPHOTO.COM/ROBERT SIMON

Always keep a message pad handy at reception

Handling information in a confidential way

Certain circumstances and situations need special care and attention and probably the most important aspect of professional communication is **confidentiality**. During our day-to-day work it is possible that we come into contact with information that others consider private. It is important that you recognise these situations and handle them accordingly. This confidential information will occur in numerous ways: during routine conversation between staff or clients, and from business contacts and inquirers. Whatever the source, you must not divulge personal or potentially sensitive information to anyone.

EKU *statement*

G2 (eku1) your salon's procedures for maintaining confidentiality

G2 (eku13) the consequences of breaking confidentiality

G2 (eku16) the confidentiality requirements within the Data Protection Act

What is confidential information?

Confidential information includes:

- the contents of client's records
- client and staff personal details such as name, address and telephone number
- financial information relating to the business.

Remember

A personal conversation can also be considered confidential – it is definitely private. People tend to talk about all sorts of things when they are in the salon, and anything that you overhear must remain private.

HAIR BY LEWIS MOORE @ FRANCESCO GROUP, STREETLY, PHOTOGRAPHY BY JOHN RAWSON@TRP

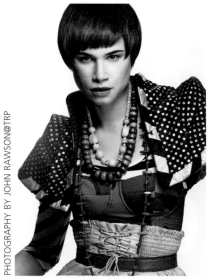

A client's confidential information is protected by law and the **Data Protection Act 1998** allows the salon to obtain, hold and use personal data, providing that the information is kept secure. The Act upholds the client's rights by preventing the unlawful disclosure of information to another person or business entity. See Appendix 1 for more information on the Data Protection Act 1998.

Remember

Personal information is private information. Never spread gossip or talk about other people's personal conversations. It's confidential!

Activity

What is your salon's/shop's policy and procedures for

1 Maintaining confidentiality?

2 Taking messages?

3 Making and recording appointments?

4 Client care at reception?

What might happen if you broke confidentiality? Write your answers in your portfolio.

G2.3 Help to make appointments for salon services

The appointment system is at the very centre of the business operation. It is essential that appointments are made accurately and promptly **every time**, whether the client makes the appointment over the telephone or comes in to the salon or shop. Before you can schedule appointments, you must have an idea of the services available. Each salon or barber's shop offers a unique "menu" of services. Different stylists or barbers will have different abilities and skills, and so might be available only for certain services at certain levels. Get to know the variety of services, the timings and costs that the salon or shop and its stylists or barbers have to offer.

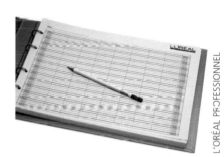

L'ORÉAL PROFESSIONNEL

The appointment system is at the very centre of the business operation

Activity

This activity is linked with the appointment system. It relates to the services and their costs at your place of work.

Service	Service abbreviation	Which stylists or barbers do this?	How long does it take?	How much does it cost?
dry cut				
wet cut				
blow dry (short hair)				
blow dry (long hair)				
shampoo and set				
"T" section highlights				
full head highlights				
roots colour				
full head colour				
permanent wave				

Remember

Always introduce yourself when handling calls. People like to speak to people they can associate with, not with strangers or machines!

Remember

Never hurry a phone call for an appointment. Rushed call handling is poor communication, rude, and will lead to making mistakes in the booking.

Remember

Never leave callers hanging on the line for more than a few seconds without checking with them first. At best, it's frustrating, at worst; they might hang up altogether!

Dealing with requests promptly and politely

Making appointments needn't be difficult. It's about matching client requests with the time available. You want to help the customer to make the booking, while bearing in mind the time it will take and who will be providing the service.

Telephone calls

You should always remember to smile, as people can **hear** the friendliness in your voice. Now say: "Good morning/afternoon this is Head Masters hair salon. This is Hayley speaking, how can I help you?". This friendly but positive approach will immediately give a professional image of both the salon and yourself. Ideally, a telephone should ring 4 or 5 times before answering; this allows the caller, who may be new to the salon or who may be an older person, the time to compose themselves in what they want to say.

Visits in person

The most popular way for clients to contact the salon is by telephone, but clients will often call in to the salon in person to make an appointment. You need to be ready for that "drop in" spontaneous client. When someone walks into the reception, they might be feeling a little uncomfortable or uneasy. Not everyone has the confidence to walk into somewhere that they don't know or can't see into. Dispel these feelings of uncertainty by making eye contact, smiling and attending to them promptly and politely by saying: "Good morning/afternoon. How may I help you?". This immediate greeting puts them at ease and leads them into providing a response that:

- will confirm that they have a booked appointment
- shows that they haven't an appointment but would like to make one
- lets you know that they are not a client but have other reasons for calling.

These are the only possible outcomes from someone making a personal visit. With this information established you can now continue.

Accurately recording appointments

Each salon has its own system for making appointments but, generally speaking, appointment scheduling is completed in such a way as to maximise the time available with appropriate staff members. Bearing this in mind, you should always remain ready, prompt and polite in attending to the client's requests. When you have found out what the caller wants, you are ready to make the appointment by asking the following questions:

- "On what day would you like the appointment?"
- "What time do you have in mind?"
- "What would you like to have done?"
- "Which stylist is that with/would you like to see?"

Each time you ask one of the questions above, you are narrowing the possible responses to a limited range. You are leading the conversation in a controlled professional way and eliminating unnecessary information that could lead you to making a mistake. The 4 questions very quickly allow you to get to the:

- right day in the appointment system
- available times for services
- type of service required by the client
- availability of their stylist to do the job.

Now you have to work out if there is enough time to make the appointment for the client. This is often the most difficult part of making appointments, because some are just a single block of time, whereas others take multiple blocks.

For example, a booking for a hair cut or a blow dry is a single block appointment. The colour or perm appointment is more complex because these straddle other appointments to allow for the colour or perm to develop, allowing the stylist to do something else in between.

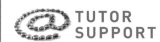

TUTOR SUPPORT

Short answer tests

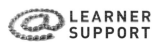

LEARNER SUPPORT

Reception puzzle

Date: Friday 13th September

Time	Clare	Steve
9.00		
9.15		
9.30	Taylor BD	
9.45		
10.00		
10.15		
10.30		

In this example we see a single block appointment made by a regular client on **Friday 13th September** at **9.30** with **Clare** for **Mrs. Taylor** for a **blow dry**

Date: Friday 13th September

Time	Clare	Steve
9.00	Summers HLT	
9.15	0123 456789	
9.30	Taylor BD	
9.45		
10.00	Summers CBD	
10.15		
10.30		

Here we see an additional appointment with contact details made on **Friday 13th September** at **9.00** with **Clare** for Miss **Summers** for a **highlights "T" section**, which now straddles the Taylor appointment and is booked back with Clare to do a cut and blow dry at 10.00

Activity

Roleplay making appointments with your colleagues. Ask your supervisor if you can use the salon's/shop's appointment system to make the test bookings. Working with your colleague, take it in turns to make appointments (in pencil) both for callers on the telephone and in person. Make a range of appointments covering a variety of services. When you have finished get your supervisor to check that you have completed the information correctly.

Appointment details

Make sure that when the booking is made that you record the information accurately and clearly and that you have considered all the factors:

- date and time
- service required
- stylist required
- the client's name
- client contact details.

EKU statement

G2 (eku5) the person in your salon to whom you should refer reception problems

Requesting assistance when needed

When you are not sure, it is always better to ask someone else than to make an incorrect booking. Some appointments are fairly straightforward, whereas others may involve some complex scheduling or assistance from the stylist involved. If you are in any doubt, go and ask the stylist involved. They will know by looking at the client's hair how long they will need to complete the work.

Sometimes the client will need a consultation prior to the appointment, say for extensions or "hair-up". These types of appointments require the stylist to have particular materials to complete the work and they may not be in stock, so will need to be ordered.

Difficult or angry clients

There may be other situations where you have to find someone else in authority to handle the client's enquiry. If you can see by a client's face (by their expressions) that they are not happy about something, it is not your job to try sort out their problem. Simply ask them to take a seat and then find a senior member of staff to deal with their concerns.

Remember

Always make sure that there are pencils, pens and eraser or correction fluid at the desk. Alterations to appointments happen all the time and you need to make those changes right away: don't leave it until later or it might not get done.

Remember

When clients arrive in person, look to see that they are nodding when you confirm the appointment details. This will show that they understand what you are saying.

Confirming and recording details correctly

Record the client's name clearly in the appointment system alongside the requested service, and check that it is scheduled for the correct day and time with the appropriate stylist. As a matter of customer service, it is also useful to give the client an approximate idea of service cost and length of appointment time. At the end, summarise all the information back to the client. This will ensure that all the details are correct.

If the client has come in to the salon or shop to make the appointment, give them an appointment card as a token of good service and as a prompt. This provides a physical copy of the appointment and another way of ensuring that all the facts are correct.

Activity
Self assessment

Don't attempt this activity until you have had some experience at reception work. Use the checklist below to self-assess. Ask your supervisor to check your responses.

Task	I do this well	I do this OK	I can't do this yet	Supervisor's comment
answering the telephone				
dealing with enquiries				
making appointments				
keeping reception clean				
restocking retail products				
restocking stationery items				

Checkerboard	I know how to keep reception clean and how to restock the displays and stationery ☐	I know how to record accurate information for messages and appointments ☐	I always follow the salon's/ shop's policy in respect to client care and customer service ☐
I know who I can turn to if I have any difficulties at work ☐	I know who to turn to for help with reception duties ☐	I understand the extent to which the Data Protection Act affects what I do at work ☐	I always carry out working practices according to the salon's policy ☐
I know how to communicate effectively with staff and customers ☐	I understand the implications of poor client communication ☐	I know how to say things in different ways in order to be tactful and courteous ☐	I understand the necessity of personal presentation when dealing with clients ☐
I know the salon's/shop's services; how long they take and how much they cost ☐	I know what to look for in relation to stationery shortages and product imperfections ☐	I understand my job and the impact of not keeping information confidential ☐	

Revision questions

Q1 Fill in the blank: All customer information and data is _____ information.

Q2 The reception should be clean and attractive throughout the working day. True or false?

Q3 Which of the following are not reception duties? (You may choose more than one answer.)

1 cleaning the product displays   4 tidying the roller trolleys

2 replenishing the till rolls   5 refilling the shampoos

3 making appointments   6 answering the telephone

Q4 If stock is delivered to reception you should always try to move it. True or false?

Q5 Which of the following should be offered to a client who arrives a little late for their appointment? (Choose one answer.)

A an alternative appointment time   C an alternative service

B a seat and a drink whilst they are waiting   D a complimentary product for home use

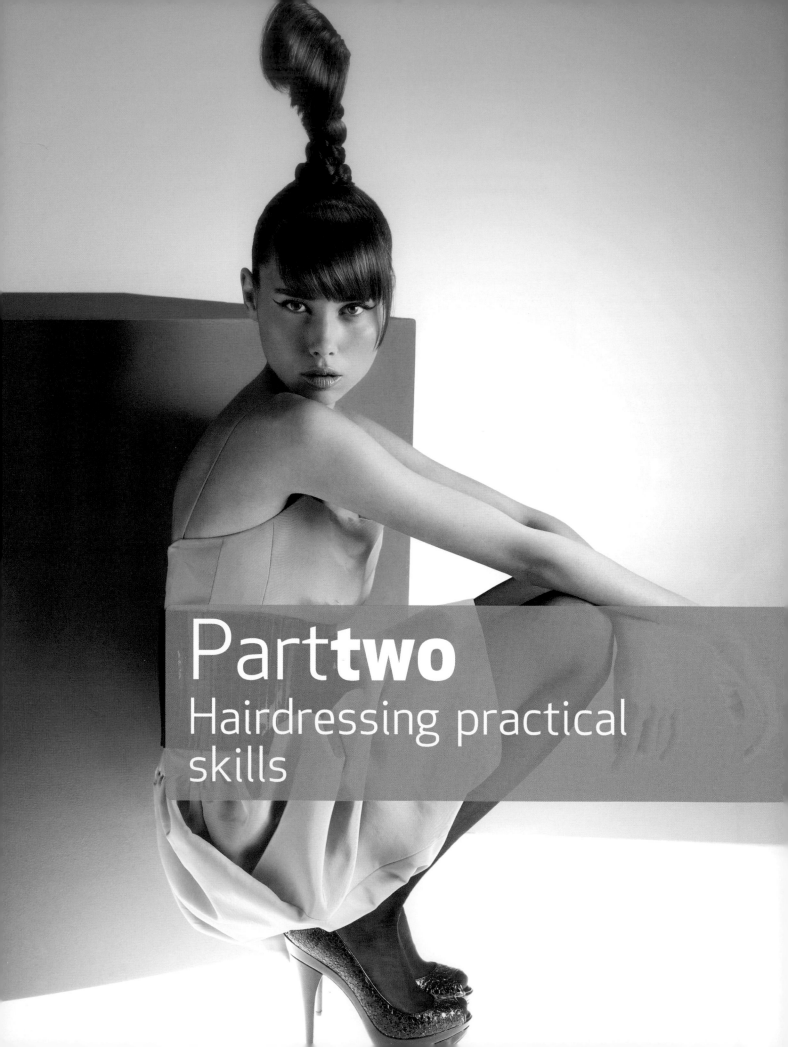

Parttwo
Hairdressing practical skills

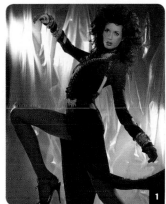

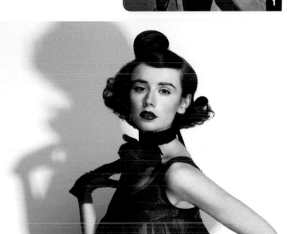

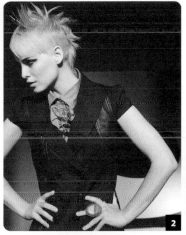

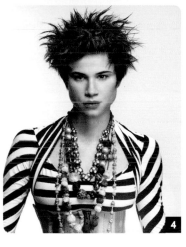

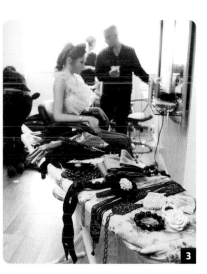

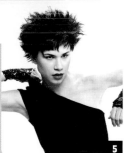

1 Hair: Richard Ward, Photography: Daniele Cipriani 2 Hair by: Damien Carney for Joico, Photography: Hama Sanders 3 Hair: NHF Inspire, Photography: Simon Powell 4 Hair by: Lewis Moore @ Francesco Group, Streetly, Photography by: John Rawson @ trp 5 Hair by: The Artistic Team @ TPL Hairdressing, Photography by: John Rawson @ trp 6 Hair by: Christopher Appleton @ George's Hair Salon, Leicester, Photography by: John Rawson @ TRP **Left** Hair by Reds Hair and Beauty, Sunderland, Photography by John Rawson @ TRP

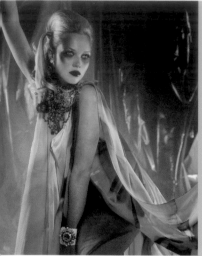

HAIR: RICHARD WARD, PHOTOGRAPHY: DANIELE CIPRIANI

Chapter**four**
Prepare for hair services and maintain work areas

GH3

GH3.1

GH3.2

CREDIT VALUE FOR UNIT GH3
2 Credits

Unit title

GH3 Prepare for hair services and maintain work areas

This is a **mandatory** unit for Level 1. It is made up of 2 main outcomes.

Main outcomes

GH3 (eku1) Prepare for hair services

GH3 (eku2) Maintain the work area for hair services

Unit GH3: quick overview

What do I need to do for GH3.1?

Carry out the following **preparations** for services:

- set up materials, tools and equipment
- make sure the stylist's tools are ready and safe to use
- get the client's records ready

What do I need to do for GH3.2?

Carry out the following **maintenance** within the salon/shop:

- dispose of waste materials
- check and clean the salon equipment
- prepare enough towels for the day
- refill and replenish low levels of salon stock
- replace the salon's resources correctly
- clean working surfaces properly so that they are ready for use

What things do I need to know?

You need to **know and understand**:

- your salon's procedures for preparation and maintenance
- your salon's procedures for the disposal of waste items
- your responsibilities in respect to COSHH
- why salons keep records
- how The Data Protection Act affects client records
- how to clean the salon's work areas

- how to set up materials, tools and equipment
- why it is important to maintain standards in hygiene and the different methods of disinfecting and sterilisation
- how to check and clean the salon's equipment
- how and where to store materials and equipment

Introduction

The salon or barber's shop environment must be kept clean and tidy at all times. The business has a duty to safeguard the health and safety of everyone who enters this space and you play an important part in helping this to take place. You and the other staff contribute to providing a safe, hygienic place through the routine duties that you perform throughout your working day. Support the stylists and barbers in their work by:

- preparing the salon/barber's shop materials, tools and equipment
- maintaining the salon/barber's shop's:
  - work surfaces
  - basins
  - floors
  - seating
  - styling units
- finding the client's records for them
- clearing up and checking after they have finished the services.

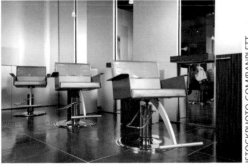

ISTOCKPHOTO.COM/RANPLETT

Your role includes keeping the salon clean and tidy

All of these basic things may seem routine, but unless they are done properly, we will be both putting our clients at risk from cross-infection or cross-infestation from poor sanitation, and putting our clients off by an untidy, unprofessional salon/barber's shop.

EKU *statement*

GH3 (eku10) how to set up materials, tools and equipment for the hair services offered by your salon

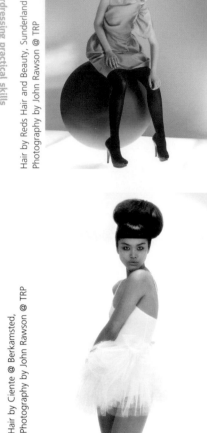

Hair by Reds Hair and Beauty, Sunderland
Photography by John Rawson @ TRP

Hair by Ciente @ Berkamsted,
Photography by John Rawson @ TRP

Set up materials, tools and equipment

As a professional, you must make sure that you are ready to provide the services to the clients at the time that they have arranged. That means that the stylists must be ready to start at the appointed time. You can't wait for people to turn up then think about what you need to do – you have to make sure that you have anticipated what will be needed and have made the necessary preparations for the following:

- perming rods, end papers, tensioning strips, setting rollers, neck wool and barrier cream are ready in the trolley trays
- brushes and combs are sterilised and ready for use
- colouring materials, bowls, brushes, foils or meshes are available
- gowns and towels are washed, clean and fresh
- hand dryers and heated equipment are ready for use at the styling units

Everything has to run to time in the salon or barber's shop; the stylists or barbers need to think about what they are going to do and you need to think about the things they might need. Most things are prepared far in advance of the time that they will be needed. For example, gowns and towels are in continual use. Salons and barber's shop usually have more than they would use on one day so that they can make laundry processes cost effective. On the other hand, a salon or shop wouldn't normally have heated tongs or straighteners for every senior member of staff. This is due in part to the likelihood that not everyone will need the same pieces of equipment at the same time, and partly because many stylists may use their own items of equipment. In either event, it doesn't matter who the equipment belongs to: if it is used within the salon it has to be made ready and safe for use.

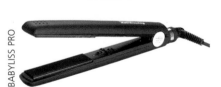

BABYLISS PRO

Think ahead: will tongs or straighteners be required for the service?

EKU statement

GH3 (eku1) your salon's requirements for work area preparation and maintenance, including the checking and cleaning of equipment

GH3 (eku9) the types of products, materials, tools and equipment required for hair services offered by your salon

Activity
Next, think about what you need to do when you arrive at work.
What things are you expected to do when you arrive at work?

....
....
....

Remember

There are always things to do in the salon
If you are not doing anything, why not get the perm rods out and check the rubbers to see if any have perished? Replace damaged, weakened or overstretched rubbers with new ones. Or you could take the curlers and rods out of the trolley trays and give them a good clean. While you are doing this, don't forget to do the trays as well!

Activity

Your salon will have its own procedures for getting things ready. Check with your supervisor how you should prepare these items then complete the activity by filling in the table below with the missing information.

Salon materials	Where are these kept?	How are they cleaned and prepared?	How long will it take to prepare?
setting rollers			
perm rods			
tensioning strips			
brushes			
combs			
colouring bowls and brushes			
gowns, towels and cutting collars			

You can see from the activity that these preparations take time. It would be unprofessional to wait for the client to arrive before doing them. Now for each of the listed items, answer the following questions.

1 What would happen if these preparations weren't carried out beforehand?

2 What could happen if they weren't done at all?

Trolleys and trays

The first job of the day, and one that always needs to be done, is sorting out and preparing the trolley trays. Because of the ways in which they can be used their contents may need to be changed several times a day.

Perm curlers are colour-coded in size order, and it is easier for the stylist to ask for a tray to be made up of red/blue and blue/grey curlers than some large ones and some smaller. But before these can be dispensed, they must be thoroughly washed and scrubbed in hot soapy water to remove all traces of perming chemicals. After washing, they need to be dried thoroughly and any broken or weak rubbers should be replaced.

Setting rollers and fabric self-cling rollers are also colour-coded in size order. These can also be washed, scrubbed and dried in a similar way to perming curlers and placed in a UV cabinet.

Colouring materials, such as bowls and brushes need to be washed and scrubbed and can be placed in a UV cabinet when they have been dried. The stylist will tell you the different lengths of foils or meshes that they need.

Salon pins, grips, etc. are easily spilled and it is very wasteful to throw them away, but if they have been on the floor they cannot be used because of the risk of cross-infection. (See the section on sterilising, page 56.)

But just cleaning the trolleys in the morning is not enough. Salon trolleys are used as multipurpose workstations throughout the day and the stylists will be using them when

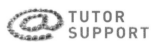
TUTOR SUPPORT

Task 4.1 Discuss preparation of the work area

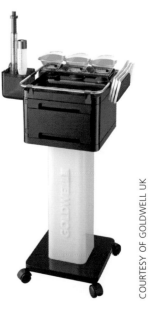
COURTESY OF GOLDWELL UK

It is your job to clean and prepare the trolleys throughout the day

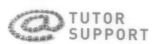

TUTOR SUPPORT

Task 4.2 List: How to help the day run smoothly

EKU *statement*

GH3 (eku8) why it is important to maintain standards of hygiene and the principles for avoiding cross-infection and cross-infestation

GH3 (eku11) methods of sterilisation and the various types of equipment available (e.g. autoclave, UV radiation, chemical sterilisation)

GH3 (eku13) the difference between sterilising and disinfecting

Remember

 Take all possible precautions to avoid dermatitis – use protective disposable gloves whenever possible. (See Chapter 1, page 12, for more information.)

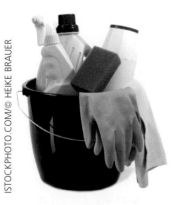

PPE is not just for salon chemicals: many cleaning solutions can also contribute to dermatitis

setting hair, blow drying, tinting and perming. With all this use, trolleys tend to need cleaning and tidying several times during the day. Fortunately they are designed with easy cleaning in mind and a simple disinfecting spray cleaner and cleaning cloth will do the job.

Make sure the stylist's tools are ready and safe to use

Hygiene and safety are the most important factors for any maintenance of tools and equipment and in Chapter 1 we covered those hazards to health and safety that can easily be seen and rectified.

However, some hazards cannot be seen, although they create equally important risks to personal health and, like the visible hazards, their impact must be minimised or eliminated.

A warm, humid salon can offer a perfect home for disease-carrying bacteria. If bacteria can find food in the form of dust and dirt, they can reproduce rapidly. Good ventilation provides a circulating current of air that will help to prevent the growth of bacteria. This is why it is important to keep the salon clean, dry and well aired at all times. This includes work areas, tools and all salon equipment.

Sterilisation

Every salon and barber's shop uses some form of sterilising system to keep the tools and equipment hygienically safe. See Chapter 1, page 15, for the required information about sterilisation.

Science

 We all carry large numbers of micro-organisms inside us, on our skin and in our hair. These organisms – **bacteria**, fungi and viruses – are too small to be seen with the naked eye. Bacteria and fungi can be seen through a microscope, but viruses are too small even for that.

Many micro-organisms are quite harmless, but some can cause disease. Those that are harmful to people are called **pathogens**. Flu, for example, is caused by a virus; athlete's foot by a fungus and skin infections like impetigo by bacteria. Conditions like these, which can be transmitted from one person to another, are said to be infectious.

Activity

How is it done where you are?

Write down your salon's methods for sterilising the tools and equipment in your salon and for disinfecting the working surfaces and basins in your salon. Write your answers in your portfolio.

Get the client's records ready

A salon or barber's shop keeps records of the services and treatments that the stylists provide to their clients. The records provide a way of maintaining details of treatments, tests and services that have been provided and continuity in future services should staffing arrangements change. These records may be kept on record cards or electronically on a computer.

The client's records are confidential and should always be handled with care. It is very easy for this information to be left around and fall into the wrong hands. For example, imagine if a client was overheard saying that all her family was just about to go on holiday for two weeks and their details (address, etc.) were left out in the salon. Anyone could see this information and use it maliciously!

EKU *statement*

GH3 (eku5) the importance of and reasons for keeping records of hair services

GH3 (eku6) the importance of the correct storage of client records in relation to the Data Protection Act

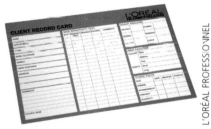

Do not ever let clients see each other's record cards

Finding treatment records

In the past, salons created simple client records for keeping service history and contact details. Traditionally, these were kept in card-index filing systems, but with the growing need to keep more information at hand, many salons now use a computer database. This is far more useful than the old card-index system because computers can find information very quickly. The way in which they search for data enables:

- easy updating and changing of information
- more information to be collected and held on file
- patterns of information to be recognised
- secure, discreet ways of keeping personal data.

The information kept by salons on computer is confidential and must be handled appropriately. The **Data Protection Act 1998** protects the clients from unlawful mishandling or breaches of security by the person accessing the information. (See Appendix 2 for more on the Data Protection Act 1998.)

Keeping client records up to date is essential because out-of-date information is useless. So when you get the records for your stylist's client, remember to check the details

EKU *statement*

GH3 (eku2) your salon's and legal requirements for the disposal of waste materials

GH3 (eku7) general salon hygiene principles in relation to floors and seating, working surfaces, mirrors and salon equipment

GH3 (eku14) how to dispose of waste materials and products from hair services

L'ORÉAL PROFESSIONNEL

such as address, telephone and mobile numbers with the client, so that the barber shop's or salon's records can be kept up to date, and that you find the right record – many people can share the same last name.

GH3.2 Maintain the work area for hair services

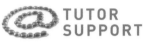

TUTOR SUPPORT

Task 4.3 List: Sterilisation

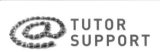

TUTOR SUPPORT

Task 4.4 Disposal of waste chart

Dispose of waste materials

The disposal of waste materials is controlled by the law. This section covers the sorts of waste that you may encounter at work.

Activity

Ask your supervisor what the arrangements are in your salon for the safe disposal of waste and **sharps**. Write your answers in your portfolio.

1 What are your salon's requirements for disposing of waste?

2 Are there any local bye-laws affecting your salon and the way that it disposes of waste?

General salon waste

The everyday items of salon waste, such as hair clippings, used colouring products, neck wool, disposable capes, etc. should be placed in an enclosed swing-lid waste bin fitted with a suitably resistant polyethylene bin liner. When the bin is full, the liner can be removed from the bin and sealed using a wire tie. Place the sealed bag in the designated area or bins ready for refuse collection. If for any reason the bin liner punctures, put the damaged liner and waste inside a second bin liner. Wash out the inside of the swing bin itself with hot water and detergent.

Activity

Preventing contamination and cross-infection is an important aspect of general health and safety. Link the statements on the left with those on the right.

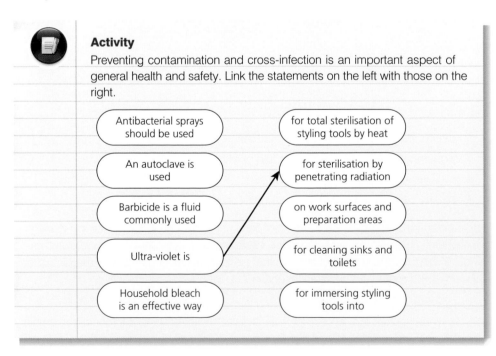

Unused, leftover colour or lightener should be washed out of colouring bowls as soon as the stylist has finished the service. These products swell up if left for any period of time and therefore need to be washed away sooner rather than later, as they might increase the risk of blocking the drains.

Disposal of used razor blades or similar sharp items

Used razor blades and similar items should be placed into the **sharps box**. See Chapter 1, page 11, for more information on the disposal of sharps.

Control of Substances Hazardous to Health (COSHH) Regulations (2002)

Your employer is required by law to consider the potential hazards to people exposed to substances within the workplace. This includes making an assessment of all substances for hazards and for those that are hazardous, either considering the use of alternative, less hazardous substances or if not, setting up procedures for safe working use. See Appendix 1 for more information about the Control of Substances Hazardous to Health (COSHH) Regulations 2002. Each local authority has its own policy on how to deal with salon waste.

EKU statement

GH3 (eku4) your own responsibilities under the current Control of Substances Hazardous to Health Regulations when handling hair products and cleaning, disinfecting and sterilising products

EKU statement

GH3 (eku16) how and where to store materials, tools and equipment

EKU statement

GH3 (eku15) how to check and clean equipment used for hair services

Activity

Complete this activity by filling in the missing information in the table below. Write your answers in your portfolio.

Salon items	Where are they kept in your salon?	How are they stored in your salon?
gowns and towels		
heated styling equipment		
salon styling products		
retail stock items		
basin/backwash products		
colour materials		

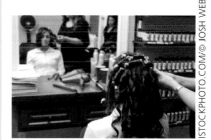

Clients will see anything dirty, murky or smeary on mirrors

Check and clean the salon equipment

Styling mirrors

Glass mirrors should always be sparkling clean! Clients sit in front of the mirrors for long periods of time, so they will definitely see those murky smears. The mirrors need to be done every morning before clients arrive and throughout the day using a window spray cleaner; this will remove all the dirt, dust and hairspray quickly.

Remember

 Hairdressers are very sensitive about their scissors: they are a stylist's most important tool. They are expensive and easily damaged if dropped! Always leave the maintenance of stylists' scissors to the stylist.

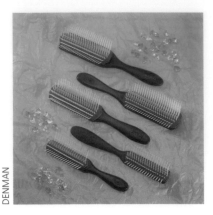

DENMAN

Plastic brushes must be washed, dried and placed in a UV cabinet for sterilising

Remember

 Always wear non-latex disposable gloves provided by the salon when cleaning salon surfaces and equipment or washing tools.

They will protect your hands from chemicals coming into contact with your skin.

Remember

Don't put contaminated items on work surfaces because they could spread infection.

Styling tools

Combs, brushes and curlers are made from hygienic, easy-to-clean plastics. Combs and brushes should be washed daily. If any styling tools are accidentally dropped on to the floor, they should not be used until they have been re-cleaned.

After washing, the dried brushes and comb can then be placed in a UV cabinet for sterilising.

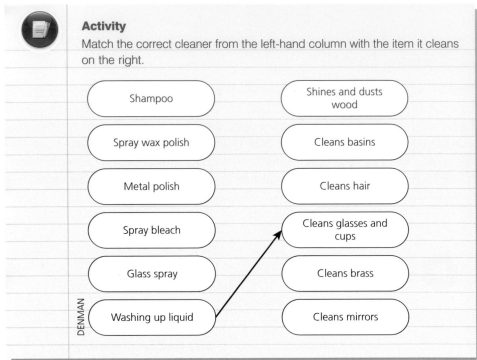

Activity

Match the correct cleaner from the left-hand column with the item it cleans on the right.

Shampoo	Shines and dusts wood
Spray wax polish	Cleans basins
Metal polish	Cleans hair
Spray bleach	Cleans glasses and cups
Glass spray	Cleans brass
Washing up liquid	Cleans mirrors

DENMAN

More and more salons use simple, work-top chemical sterilising jars. These are an efficient way of cleaning implements hygienically between clients, but remember to make sure that the tools are rinsed before use because they have been immersed in to strong chemicals. (See the section on sterilisation in Chapter 1 on page 15.)

Hood dryers, colour accelerators and steamers

Hood dryers, colour accelerators and steamers are made out of tough vinyl mouldings over metal frames. They all run by electricity and should therefore be handled and cleaned with extreme care (see Chapter 1, page 15). Spray cleaners produce the best results because they expel the minimum amount of cleaning fluid, which helps to prevent product dripping into the equipment. This could cause it to malfunction or short-out.

Daily dusting and cleaning is normally done at the beginning and periodically throughout the day. When an item of equipment is used, say for a colour service, make sure that the equipment is checked and wiped immediately after use. This will ensure that other clients are not exposed to any hazards, and that the machinery is defaced or stained.

A steamer is used for bleaching processes. It looks like a portable hood dryer with a water tank reservoir on the top. The water tank is removable and can be filled with tap water; the tank is replaced into the machine and a heating element boils the water when

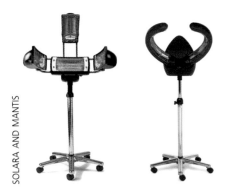

SOLARA AND MANTIS

Use spray cleaners to clean electric items like this

it is switched on. As the water boils inside the machine, the steam is transferred to the twin-walled, transparent hood part of the steamer. A series of small holes inside the inner wall of the steamer allows steam to emerge and provide a hot, moist heat, which is delivered to the person seated beneath. **Always wait for the equipment too cool down before cleaning or replacing it.**

Basin/backwash areas

Basins have ceramic finishes, which are hard wearing but brittle. Never put metal, ceramic or glassware items into them because they could crack or be damaged. General cleaning should take place at the beginning of the day, although they will need routine checking and cleaned every time they are used. This is particularly noticeable around the basin's neck area, especially after clients have had colouring or bleaching services. Simple spray cleaners containing bleach are an ideal, hygienic solution for both the bowl and chrome mixer valves as they minimise the possibility of cross-infection or cross-infestation. Make sure that the **hair traps** are replaced because these stop loose hairs going down drains and causing blockages, which could be both disruptive and expensive to put right.

Prepare enough towels for the day

Every client should have a clean, fresh towel and gown. These are an essential part of the daily salon equipment and busy salons and barber's shops tend to get through mountains of towels on a daily basis. So get to know how to use the salon's washing machine and tumble dryer. These will be in constant use and a quick turn around of laundry will be expected.

Refill and replenish low levels of salon stock

Products need replacing on a daily basis. It's not good enough to leave things that need replacing for another day, or for someone else to do it because other staff will not be able to use the correct products on their clients and sales will be lost unless sold retail items are replaced on the shelves.

Basins are in continual use, and as clients are shampooed and conditioned, the products run down. Salons use a lot of different shampoos and conditioners. Unlike the shampoos that you can buy from the supermarket, the salon buys its products in bulk sizes. Each type of shampoo and conditioner used by the salon at the backwash area is contained in large pump dispensers. When a product runs out, the correct product must be refilled into the backwash size as soon as possible. The large bulk sizes are usually kept away from the salon floor in the stock area. You should ask for permission to take the basin size containers away for refilling.

Carefully match the bulk sizes to the ones needing refilling. For each one, undo the screw top and clean the pump. Then, using a funnel, carefully top up the product to just below the neck. If you overfill, you could waste product when you try to replace the pump. After filling the container, wipe up any spills and replace the bulk containers back into storage. You can then take the refills back to the basins.

Other products will be in continual use as stylists work on their clients. Keep checking up on salon styling materials, so that they don't run out. If you notice that a product is

Remember

 Electrical tools and equipment should be subjected to a portable appliance test (PAT) and checked by a qualified person each year.

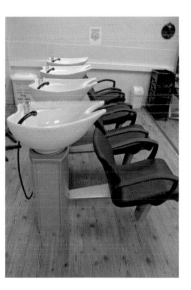

Basins need to be checked and cleaned after each use with spray bleach cleaner

Remember

 Always ask your supervisor what you can put down the basins. Never pour anything down the drain unless you know that it is safe.

Remember

 Gowns should be machine washed to remove perfume, body odours or staining and to prevent the spread of cross-infection or cross-infestation.

EKU *statement*

GH3 (eku3) your salon's required stocking levels for products and other items used in hair services

Remember

 Wipe up any spills on work surfaces or floors as this could be a hazard to someone else: they could slip.

Remember

 The barber's shop and hair salon is a public place and should always be clean and appealing. You have an important part to play in its overall success. Remember – a tidy salon is easier to clean, so get into the habit of clearing work areas as you go along.

EKU *statement*

GH3 (eku12) how to clean, disinfect and sterilise different types of tools for the different hair services (i.e. metals, plastic, wood, electrical)

GH3 (eku12) the condition in which the work area should be left ready for further services

getting low, don't throw it away. Instead, ask the stylist if you should go and get a replacement out of stock ready, for when it runs out.

Retail displays in reception are an expensive investment for the salon and stock resting on shelves is an expensive cost. Products provide a useful, additional input to the barber shop's or salon's income and many shops and salons look for a significant proportion of their turnover to be derived from these sales. As product sales from reception are an extremely important **revenue stream** for the salon or shop; you can help the receptionist by keeping the stocks refilled. During the day, retail products will run down and will need replacing. You should ask permission to go and find the correct replacements so that the stock levels can be maintained. Always make a point of dusting the existing products on the shelf because no-one will want to handle or buy dusty items. Retail displays should invite clients to browse; they prompt clients to ask questions or ask for advice.

Most hair products have a long shelf life, that is, they will not perish or deteriorate over time like food products do. But as a routine way of selling older products first, it is normal practice to put the newer replacements at the back of the shelves and bring the older ones to the front. This system is called **stock rotation** and is a generally accepted practice.

Replace the salon's resources correctly

Always put something back after it has been used so that it can be found next time it is needed – equipment that is not put away can also be a hazard. Each client deserves the best possible service and you can help by putting things away so that they are ready for next time. Hand dryers and heated equipment should be put back in their proper place for safety. Trailing leads need to be carefully coiled so that they don't present a hazard to the next user. Trolleys should be removed, and their items cleaned and trays re-organised. Tools need to be cleaned and products put back tidily.

Activity

Find out what your barber shop's or salon's procedures are for replenishing low levels of:

● basin/backwash items

● styling products at the work stations

● retail products on display shelving in the reception area

Activity

Think about cleaning

Look at the list below and then fill in the missing information for how it should be cleaned and how often it should be done. Write your answers in your portfolio.

Salon area	How should this be cleaned?	How often should it be done?
work surfaces		
glass and mirrors		
carpets and working area floors		
wash basins		

Clean working surfaces properly so that they are ready for use

Clean the work areas (reception, workstations, backwash and stock preparation areas) – this means dusting and/or washing-down at least once each day. Fortunately, salons and barber's shops tend to have easy-to-wipe surfaces made of plastic, glass, tiles or lacquered wood.

When clients have been finished, the styling sections need to be put ready for use again. This isn't left for the end of the day because the styling sections are in continual use and no-one wants to sit in someone else's hair clippings or left-behind debris. You need to clear the working surfaces of tools, cups and saucers, magazines etc. The sections can be cleaned with spray surface cleaner or hot water and detergent, then dried and wiped free of smears so that they look shiny and appealing.

Salon floors and seating

The floors should be kept clean at all times. This means that they will need regular mopping, sweeping or vacuuming, particularly following periods of wet weather when dirt is "tracked in" from outside. When a work area is mopped, make sure that other staff (or clients) are aware that the area is wet and may be slippery. When using the vacuum cleaner, make a point of checking the collection bag and filters. It doesn't take long for hair clippings to fill the bag. This impairs the vacuum's ability to clean properly.

It is much easier to see that vinyl or ceramic floor coverings need cleaning than it is to see that a floor covered in carpet is dirty. If floors need mopping and cleaning, try to do this at a quieter time of the day, probably at the end of the working day so they can dry out totally overnight. If spillages happen during the day it will be necessary to mop up during times when clients are in the salon. When this does occur, make sure that any wet or damp areas are dried immediately afterwards because this will minimise the chance of anyone slipping.

Most salons buy in industrial cleaning products for routine maintenance. These products come in bulk sizes and are far more appropriate for deep, hygienic cleaning than their retail counterparts. Know exactly what each product does. More often than not, these products will need to be diluted before use. Always read the manufacturers' instructions before use and remember to wear the correct personal protective equipment (PPE). After mopping or waxing floors, dispose of residual fluids by the shop's or salon's designated method. Clean the mop thoroughly, rinse well and wring it out before putting it back into store.

Salon styling chairs   Salon styling chairs are made of durable, easy-to-clean materials. Because they are in constant use, the backs of the chairs will often be over-sprayed with hairspray. These should be washed or sponged regularly with hot water and detergent. Don't leave them wet; dry them off with a towel. The bases of styling chairs need cleaning too; most chairs have a solid or "5-point star" metal or vinyl base. These should be dusted and cleaned at least once a day and washed at least once a week. Chairs with a hydraulic lift have solid bases, like the classic barber's chair, and are heavier – normally a metal alloy or chrome. They need cleaning every day with a suitable spray, followed by a "buffing" and polishing.

Remember

Clear up spillages immediately. If you don't know what was spilled, ask someone for assistance.

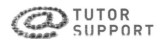

TUTOR SUPPORT

Task 4.6 List: Product replenishment, storage and handling

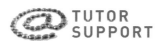

TUTOR SUPPORT

Task 4.5 List: Salon environment

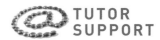

TUTOR SUPPORT

Short answer tests

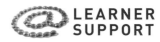

LEARNER SUPPORT

Preparing for services puzzle

Checkerboard

	I know my salon's work preparation routines ☐	I know my salon's policy in respect to disposing of waste materials and products ☐	I know how to check product levels and refill when necessary ☐
I understand my salon's client record systems and the importance of confidentiality ☐	I know what things to use for keeping the salon areas hygienically clean and safe ☐	I understand how cross-infection and cross-infestation occur and how to prevent it ☐	I know the methods of sterilisation ☐
I know how to sterilise the various materials used for styling at work ☐	I know the methods of disinfecting ☐	I can handle, use and work with materials, products and equipment safely ☐	I know where materials and equipment is kept at work ☐

Revision questions

Q1 Fill in the blank: Clients should never be put at risk from cross-infection or cross _____.

Q2 Sterilisation kills all living organisms. True or false?

Q3 Which of the following should be sterilised in an autoclave? (You may choose more than one answer.)

1) brushes   4) scissors
2) combs   5) clipper blades
3) sectioning clips 6) used razor blades

Q4 Disinfectants kill all living organisms. True or false?

Q5 Which of the following is a form of chemical sterilisation? (Choose one answer.)

A UV cabinet   C Barbicide™
B autoclave   D disinfectant spray

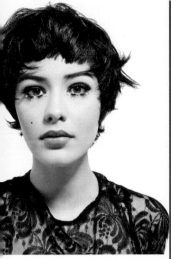

HAIR: TERRY CALVERT & THE CLIPSO ARTISTIC TEAM

GH1

GH1.1
GH1.2
GH1.3

CREDIT VALUE FOR UNIT GH1
4 Credits

Unit title

GH1 Shampoo and condition hair

This is a **mandatory** unit for Level 1. It is made up of 3 main outcomes.

Main outcomes

GH1 (eku1) Maintain effective and safe methods of working when shampooing and conditioning hair

GH1 (eku2) Shampoo hair

GH1 (eku3) Apply conditioners to the hair

Chapter**five**
Shampoo and condition hair

Unit GH1: quick overview

What do I need to do for GH1.1?

You need to **prepare for shampooing and conditioning** by:

- correctly protect and position clients and yourself
- keeping the basin area clean and safe to use
- maintaining personal hygiene standards
- monitoring the levels of materials
- completing the service efficiently

What do I need to do for GH1.2?

You need to **shampoo the client's hair** by:

- types of shampoo
- following the stylist's instructions
- using the correct massage techniques
- controlling the water flow and temperature
- rinsing and finishing off

What do I need to do for GH1.3?

You need to **condition the client's hair** by:

- following the stylist's instructions
- using the appropriate technique
- rinsing and finishing off

Keywords

Anti-oxidant conditioner

stops the oxidation process of chemical services

Cross-infestation

the passing of animal parasites from one to another

Dermatitis

an occupational disease affecting the skin

Effleurage

a light stroking, shampoo massage movement applied with either the fingers or the palms of the hands

Friction

a firm, vigorous rubbing massage technique made by the fingertips, used during shampooing

Hydrophilic

water loving

Hydrophobic

water repelling

Petrissage

a kneading movement of the skin that lifts and compresses underlying structures of the skin, used when applying conditioner

pH balance

the natural acid mantle of skin and hair at pH5.5

Rotary

a quicker and firmer circulatory movement used in shampooing

Surface conditioner

a light conditioner that works on the outside of the hair to smooth and fill areas of damaged, missing or worn cuticle until next shampoo

What things do I need to cover?

You will be:

- handling different lengths of hair
- using different massage techniques
- applying surface and treatment conditioners

What things do I need to know?

You need to **know and understand:**

- your salon's way of preparing and protecting clients
- health and safety laws affecting the service
- how to maintain the basin area
- how to work safely and hygienically at all times
- the basic science relating to shampooing and conditioning
- how to use electrical equipment associated with conditioning treatments
- the problems that can occur during shampooing and conditioning and who these should be referred to
- how and when to use different massage techniques
- how to remove products from the hair and detangle after
- the importance of being cost effective

Introduction

Shampooing and conditioning is a service that forms part of many other salon processes. When done properly, this service provides a personal, invigorating and stimulating therapeutic experience that creates the initial impression of the services that are going to follow.

This is your opportunity to provide luxury

Shampooing and conditioning well can show that you not only care about your work, but want to prove that you too, are a professional part of the salon team.

What does shampooing and conditioning do?

Shampooing cleans the hair by removing dirt, grease, skin scale, sweat and product build-up, leaving the hair ready for blow drying, setting or perming.

Conditioning treatments smooth the cuticle layer, provide protection for the hair, improve handling and combing, make the hair look healthier and help the hair to resist external elements.

How do shampoos work?
Shampoos come in a variety of forms – gels, oils, creams and pastes. Some are milder and gentler on the hair than others. They need different compositions so that they can treat different hair types and conditions.

- stronger, cleansing shampoos tend to be for greasier hair types
- mild shampoos tend to be for frequent everyday use
- moisturising shampoos replenish much needed moisture and oil to dry, porous hair.

Different shampoos have different formulations, but they all contain detergent, which will remove dirt and grease. Water molecules are attracted to each other by small electrical forces. These have their greatest effect at the water's surface, creating what is called **surface tension**. On hair, water by itself would form droplets. The detergent in shampoo reduces the surface tension, allowing the water to spread easily over the hair and scalp. Each detergent molecule has two ends similar to a magnet. The **hydrophilic** end is attracted to water molecules; the other, **hydrophobic**, end repels water and is attracted to dirt and grease instead. Detergent molecules lift the grease off the hair and suspend it in the water. This suspension is called an **emulsion**. The grease holds the dirt, so as the grease is removed, the dirt loosens too. The emulsion containing the dirt is rinsed away with water, leaving the hair clean.

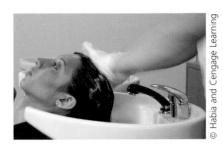
Shampooing is a luxurious, therapeutic experience

© Habia and Cengage Learning

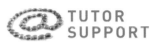
TUTOR SUPPORT

Task 5.1 Investigate what does shampooing and conditioning do

EKU *statement*

GH1 (eku17) how the build up of products can affect the hair, scalp and effectiveness of other services

EKU *statement*

GH1 (eku16) how shampoo and water act together to cleanse the hair

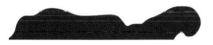

Dirt/grease on the surface of the hair

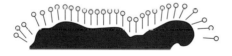

Detergent molecules attracted to dirt

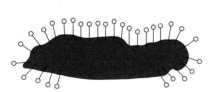

Detergent attaches itself all around the dirt breaking the surface tension, bonding it to the surface of the hair

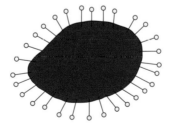

Detergent encapsulates the dirt, removing it from the surface of the hair; suspended in an emulsion

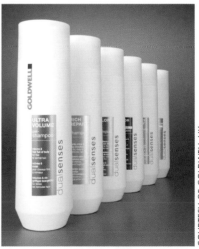
COURTESY OF GOLDWELL UK

Shampoos come in different formulations for different hair types and conditions

How do conditioners work?
Conditioners provide a variety of benefits for hair. They can create a protective barrier that reduces the damage caused by sunlight, drying

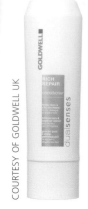
COURTESY OF GOLDWELL UK

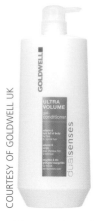
COURTESY OF GOLDWELL UK

Conditioners provide a variety of benefits to different types of hair

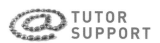
TUTOR SUPPORT

Task 5.2 Investigate how shampoos work

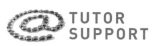
TUTOR SUPPORT

Task 5.3 Discuss - Health and safety issues

and heating. They can re-balance the hair after chemical processes and even help to strengthen and improve weakened hair. They work in two ways to provide these benefits by bonding with the hair through:

- **Absorption** – this relies upon the natural state of the hair. Dry and porous hair has many tiny spaces within the hair's internal structure. These areas suck in the conditioning agents by capillary action, just as water is drawn into a sponge.
- **Attraction** – this occurs after the hair has been shampooed. The action of the detergent on the hair during shampooing ensures that all product, dirt and dust are removed. When these particles are removed it leaves the surface of the hair in a **+charged** (positively charged) state. This prepares the hair for the conditioner, which is now attracted to the sites upon the hair that have been electrically charged.

This ionic attraction principle can be explained another way. Think of how balloons can be stuck to the wall by rubbing them vigorously on the sleeve of your jumper. This removes electrical particles and now makes the balloon stick to anything it comes into contact with, just like a magnet!

EKU statement

GH1 (eku1) your salon's requirements for client preparation

GH1 (eku4) your own responsibilities under the current Control of Substances Hazardous to Health Regulations in relation to the use of shampoos and conditioning products

GH1 (eku7) the range of protective clothing that should be available to clients

GH1 (eku8) how the position of your client and yourself can affect the desired outcome and reduce fatigue and the risk of injury

GH1 (eku9) the safety considerations which must be taken into account when shampooing and conditioning

GH1.1 Maintain effective and safe methods of working when shampooing and conditioning hair

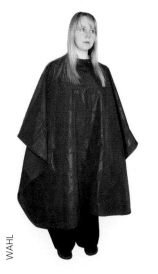
WAHL

The gown protects the client's clothes

Correctly protect and position clients and yourself

The client's clothes must be protected from spills and splashes with a clean, freshly laundered gown with a fresh, clean towel placed around the shoulders and fixed with a sectioning clip. Watch the towel in relation to the basin and the client's neck when you shampoo or condition. If there isn't enough towel between the basin and neck, water can seep down the client's neck and wet their clothes. Too much fabric will soon become saturated, making the client uncomfortable and wetting their clothes.

It is very important that, after sitting the client at the basin, you ensure that they are comfortable and that their back and neck are fully supported by the position of the seat and the basin. When the client is correctly seated, the basin forms a supportive barrier at the nape of the neck. It should neither pinch and cause discomfort, nor should it allow water to leak over the rim.

Your posture

Your standing position is equally important from a safety point of view. You should stand close enough to the basin so that you can stand upright when:

- in a **side wash position**, where your arms and shoulders are positioned above the torso and hips without twisting or leaning forwards
- or in a **back wash position**, where your arms and shoulders are directly above your hips and feet and slightly behind the position of the client's head when they lie back.

You need to maintain the same posture throughout the shampoo or conditioning process, otherwise you will be exposing yourself to the risk of injury and longer term back condition or fatigue.

Remember

Some injuries or neck complaints prevent the client from lying back at the basin. In some cases this has led to clients passing out when pressure is applied to the back of the neck. Ask your client if they know of any reason why they cannot use a backwards style wash-point.

Activity

Answer the following questions in your portfolio.

1 Why is your posture important when you are shampooing and conditioning?

2 What safety considerations do you have to think about whilst the client is at the basin?

3 Why do you have to rinse the hair well after shampooing or conditioning?

4 Why do you need to keep the wash area clean and tidy?

Keeping the basin area clean and safe to use

Remember to keep the work area clean and tidy at all times. All items should be removed from the sinks and side areas before any client sits at the basin. This will include:

- empty, waste product containers, such as conditioners or shampoos
- colouring bowls, brushes and colour products in general
- perming solutions or neutraliser in bottles or bowls, used end papers and sponges
- used neck wool, plastic caps and capes
- loose hair caught in the hair traps in the drain.

Surprisingly, all these items tend to find their way to the basin area at some point during the day, and all of them are unhygienic and pose a risk to the client's health unless they are dealt with in the appropriate way. For more information on the disposal of general salon waste, see Chapter 4, Prepare for hair services and maintain work areas, page 58.

EKU statement

GH1 (eku10) why it is important to keep your work area clean and tidy

EKU statement

GH1 (eku6) what is contact dermatitis and how to avoid developing it whilst carrying out hairdressing services

GH1 (eku11) methods of working safely and hygienically and which minimise the risk of cross-infection and cross-infestation

GH1 (eku12) the importance of personal hygiene

Maintaining personal hygiene standards

All the materials that come into contact with the client's skin must be clean and hygienic. Similarly, your own personal standards of health and hygiene should not present any risk to client either. This will prevent the risk of cross-infection and helps to maintain a healthy, safe environment. You must also take care of your hands to prevent developing **dermatitis**. Contact dermatitis is an occupational disease that can affect your hands; it creates a painful, itching sensation accompanied with a reddening and cracking of the skin.

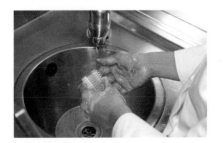

Ensure hands and nails are clean to avoid cross-infection

Remember

 Always wear non-latex disposable gloves when you handle any chemicals and follow the manufacturers' instructions.

EKU *statement*

GH1 (eku2) the person to whom you should report low levels of resources

GH1 (eku31) the importance of using shampoos and conditioners cost effectively

Remember

 Always use a funnel to top up the shampoos and conditioners at the basin. This will prevent spillage and unnecessary waste. Pouring from a 5-litre container into a narrow-necked 1-litre container is very difficult!

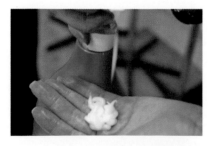

Any more than this is wasteful and would end up rinsed down the drain!

For more information on preventing infection, avoiding dermatitis and personal health and hygiene, see Chapter 1, Make sure your own actions reduce risks to health and safety, pages 12 and 20–21.

Monitoring the levels of materials

The shampoos and conditioners are in continual use at the basin area and may need refilling throughout the day. Keep checking the levels of product throughout the day. Get used to gauging the weight of a full bottle as opposed to one that is nearly empty. Don't wait until they have run out; fill them as required. When you refill a product, unscrew the pump fitting and rinse it well to remove any dried-on product.

Always use shampoo and conditioners sparingly; they are professional products so a small amount goes a long way. Un-economical use of products is a waste of material resources will reduce business profits. Most salons tend to use their shampoos and conditioners in pump action dispensers because this enables you to obtain the product without having to pick the containers up. This method is particularly helpful because you could have wet hands and the container could easily slip, or spill over the floor, the basin or the client!

Water is essential to all the salon's services, and shampooing alone can take 5–10 litres for each wash! It is vitally important that this valuable and expensive resource is not unnecessarily wasted. Make sure that you always use water sparingly and **never** leave the taps running between shampoos, even if it is "just" the cold water!

EKU *statement*

GH1 (eku3) your salon's expected service time for shampooing and conditioning

GH1 (eku13) the importance of thoroughly rinsing hair when shampooing and conditioning

GH1 (eku19) the manufacturers' instructions relating to the use of shampooing and conditioning products in your salon

GH1 (eku21) what may happen if instructions for shampooing and conditioning hair are not followed

GH1 (eku22) the types and causes of problems that can arise when shampooing and conditioning hair

GH1 (eku24) when and how to use rotary, effleurage and petrissage massage techniques when shampooing and conditioning different lengths of hair

Completing the service efficiently

Keep an eye on the clock: you must remember that all wash-point activities are part of a wider hairdressing service, and the stylist will need the client back in the styling chair as soon as possible so that they don't overrun and don't make the client late. You must do your part of the service in an acceptable timeframe that suits the salon's expected time-scales. Typically, a shampoo and simple **surface conditioner** should take 3–5 minutes.

Preparing to shampoo checklist

- prepare the client with a clean fresh gown and towel
- make sure the client is comfortable and the position of the basin is correct

- brush through the hair carefully to remove any tangles and look for any signs of infection, infestation or injury that would stop you from carrying out the service
- ask the stylist what products you should use
- get the products ready and close at hand

Remember

Always follow the manufacturers' instructions when using any chemical products.

Activity

Shampooing processes can differ between salons. What is the preferred process for shampooing in your salon, and how long should it take? Write your response in the space provided.

1

2

3

4

Remember

Hard rubbing and an uneven pressure during rotary massage are uncomfortable for the client. Practise the right pressure with your colleagues at the salon.

GH1.2   Shampoo hair

Types of shampoo

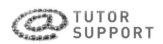

TUTOR SUPPORT

Task 5.4 List - Determine the amount of shampoo needed

There are many types of shampoo, and the table below provides you with a range of some of the most popular types and the effects that they have on hair.

Type	Effects on the hair
aloe vera	a popular, mild natural base ideal for healthy hair and scalps that can be used on a frequent basis
camomile	better on greasy hair; has a natural lightening effect
clarifying	strong, deep acting often used prior to chemical services to remove build-up of styling products and dirt
coconut	contains an emollient which helps dry hair to regain its smoothness and elasticity
jojoba	a natural base; better on normal to drier hair types
lemon	contains citric acid; ideal for greasy hair types or for removing product build-up
medicated	helps to maintain the normal state of the hair and scalp; contains antiseptics such as juniper or tea tree oil
mint	a natural base suited to normal to slightly greasy hair, often used as a frequent use shampoo
oil	can contain a range of natural bases such as pine, palm and almond; these are used to smooth and soften drier hair and scalps
soya	helps to lock in moisture for the hair and scalp
tea tree oil	a natural essential oil, which is like an antiseptic that will fight infections on the scalp

Remember

 If you have any difficulties with the shampooing and conditioning process or any equipment that you are using, ask the stylist for assistance.

Remember

 Always check with the client to make sure that the temperature is comfortable and not too hot for either piece of equipment.

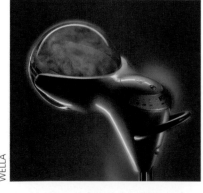

WELLA

A steamer uses moist heat to help the conditioner penetrate

Activity

To complete this activity, copy the table below into your portfolio and then for each shampoo that your salon uses at the basin, complete the missing information. Use as many rows as you need.

Shampooing product	Who is the manufacturer?	What hair type is it for?	What does the product do?

Following the stylist's instructions

For products and equipment

Choosing the right products for the type of hair and following services are very important. If the wrong shampoo is selected, the hair might become difficult to handle, fly away, static, brittle or dull. Similarly, when the hair is to be permed or coloured and the shampoo doesn't remove the styling products from the hair, they might block the action of the chemicals in the technical service and interfere with the overall expected result! For these reasons it is essential that you **ask the stylist** what products you should use. Keep them to hand throughout the process.

Some conditioning processes need heat to accelerate the beneficial action of the treatment. This can be applied by either a hood dryer or a steamer.

Hood dryer The hood dryer applies **dry heat** to the conditioning process. It will develop the treatment more quickly than if it were left at room temperature; it enables the product to penetrate more deeply into the hair, where, if it were left without heat, it might not work as well. A hood dryer will take a few minutes to reach operating temperature, so turn it on and let it heat up whilst you are shampooing.

Steamer A steamer applies **moist heat**; it looks like a portable hood dryer with a water tank reservoir on the top. The water tank is removable and can be filled with tap water; the tank is replaced into the machine and a heating element boils the water when it is switched on. As the water boils inside the machine, the steam is transferred to the twin-walled, transparent hood part of the steamer. A series of small holes within the inner wall of the steamer allows steam to emerge and provide a hot, moist heat that is delivered to the person seated beneath. Like the hood dryer, it enables the product to penetrate more deeply than if left without heat, although a steamer has the added benefit of not drying the product on the surface of the hair because the steam keeps the treatment moist. Keep an eye on the levels of water within the reservoir.

Remember

 Both the hood drier and the steamer are electrical items. Always check the condition of the plug and lead before turning it on. See Appendix 1 for more information about the Electricity at Work Regulations 1989.

Activity

Answer the following questions in your portfolio:

1 How long should it take to complete the shampoo and conditioning service at work?

2 What is dermatitis and how do you avoid contracting it?

3 What types of protective wear are available for clients while they are in the salon?

4 How would you know which shampoo to use on a client?

5 Why is it important to keep checking the water temperature during shampooing?

6 Why should you turn the water off between shampoos?

EKU *statement*

GH1 (eku17) how the build up of products can affect the hair, scalp and effectiveness of other services

GH1 (eku30) how often to shampoo and condition the hair according to hairstyle, hair and scalp condition and lifestyle

Using the correct massage techniques

The purpose of shampooing is to prepare the hair for other services. It uses a combination of techniques in order to remove dirt and grease, product build-up and skin scale. Longer hair is more difficult to handle than shorter hair, although the same techniques are used for any lengths. In general:

- longer hair often requires two shampoos in order to develop a good lather
- short hair will often lather well with just one shampoo
- oilier, greasy hair usually needs at least two shampoos because it takes longer for the detergent in the shampoo to emulsify the grease and release it from the hair
- drier hair types can often be difficult to moisten and may also need two shampoos.

The massage techniques

There are three massage techniques used in the shampooing: **effleurage**, **rotary** and **friction**; a fourth technique, **petrissage**, is used in conditioning.

Effleurage   Effleurage is a light stroking movement applied with either the fingers or the palms of the hands. It is applied with an even, rhythmical movement with very little pressure, to induce a feeling of relaxation.

Rotary   Rotary is a circulatory movement made by the fingertips and thumbs with the hands in a loose "claw like" holding position. It is applied with even pressure on either side of the head, working from the sides above the ears backwards, over the back of the head and down into the nape of the neck. The rubbing process activates the shampoo, forming a rich lather, and can be repeated until the hair is clean.

Friction   Friction is a firmer, faster rubbing action made by the fingertips with the hands, again in a loose "claw like" position. Friction is used for certain hair and scalp conditions or otherwise requested by the client for a more vigorous shampooing experience.

Remember

Wet hair can tangle easily, which makes it very painful to comb through. Therefore, when combing through wet hair, always start at the nape. Disentangle the ends first; then work back up through the lengths getting closer to the scalp.

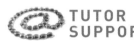
TUTOR SUPPORT

Task 5.5 Length of time to complete a shampoo and conditioning

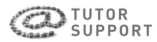
TUTOR SUPPORT

Task 5.6 List types of shampoos

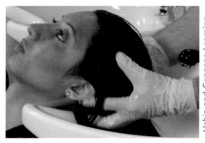
Habia and Cengage Learning

Use rotary massage technique to cleanse the hair and scalp.

TUTOR SUPPORT

Task 5.7 Shampoos used in the salon chart

Petrissage Petrissage is a kneading movement of the skin that lifts and compresses underlying structures of the skin. The pressure applied should be intermittent and light, although firm enough to invigorate the part being treated.

EKU *statement*

GH1 (eku25) how to shampoo hair and the potential consequences of doing this wrongly
GH1 (eku26) the importance of evenly distributing shampoo

Activity
You can always find out if your own shampooing practices are acceptable if you shampoo your colleagues' hair at work. Ask each other about the experience, and in what ways you need to modify or change your techniques.

Step by step: shampooing

Step 1 Sit the client at the basin, put on a clean fresh gown and visually check the hair and scalp.

Step 2 Place a freshly laundered towel around the client's neck and across their shoulders.

Step 3 Adjust the basin so that when the client's head is tilted back their position is comfortable, with the minimum of towel supporting their neck.

Step 4 When working on longer hair, carefully disentangle the hair by initially working the fingers through the lengths and then by brushing or with a wide-toothed comb.

Step 5 Turn on the water and adjust the mixture of hot and cold. Test the temperature on the back of your hand to ensure the temperature is neither too hot nor too cold.

Step 6 Carefully place your hand across the client's hairline, "damming" the water from splashing forward onto the face. Start rinsing the hair from the forehead, down either side, cupping the ears and through to the lengths.

Step 7 Check the water pressure and temperature and ask the client throughout.

Step 8 After the hair is thoroughly wet, apply a small amount of the correct shampoo to the palms of the hand; lightly rub them together, then apply evenly to the client's hair to distribute the shampoo correctly.

Step 9 With your fingers clawed, massage the scalp with the correct massage techniques. Cover the whole scalp ensuring that no part is missed.

Step 10 Rinse the hair thoroughly, checking water temperature and pressure.

Step 11 Finally, rinse all traces of shampoo lather away from the hair and lightly squeeze out the excess water so that the hair is free of lather and ready for the next process. Repeat steps 5–11 if a second shampoo is needed.

Remember

Sharp fingernails can scratch or tear the skin, causing the client discomfort and possibly infection. Keep your nails smoothly manicured.

EKU *statement*

GH1 (eku15) the effects of water temperature on the scalp

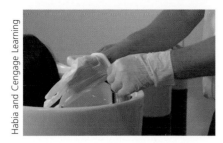

Habia and Cengage Learning

Protective gloves are worn to help prevent contact dermatitis.

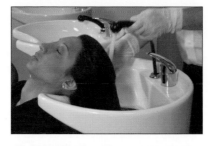

Step 5 Always check the water temperature before wetting the client's hair.

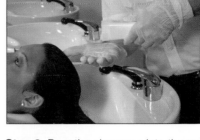

Step 8 Pour the shampoo into the palm of the hand and not directly on to the client's hair.

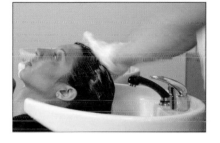

Step 8 (continued) Apply the shampoo to the hair by spreading it down the hair length using effleurage massage technique.

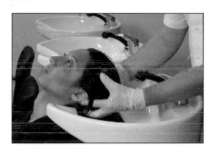

Step 9 Use rotary massage technique to cleanse the hair and scalp.

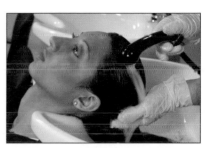

Step 11 Rinse the hair thoroughly to make sure all the shampoo has been removed from the hair and scalp. Carry out the shampoo process twice to ensure all dirt, grease and product build up is removed from the hair.

Controlling the water flow and temperature

When shampooing, control the water pressure to make sure that it is fast enough to rinse the hair properly, but slow enough so that it doesn't spray the client's face. Check the water temperature regularly by running the water over and between your fingers whilst you are rinsing. This way you will be able to gauge any fluctuations in temperature. Many water systems draw from the same water supply – other staff drawing water at the same time, and appliances elsewhere in the building, such as washing machines, toilets and sinks, can make the water temperature fluctuate at the wash-point very quickly. You need to be sensitive to those changes in temperature so that the client doesn't get burned!

EKU *statement*

GH1 (eku28) importance of removing products and excess water from the hair after each service

Remember

Always report blocked pipes or basins immediately. Standing waste water is quickly contaminated by bacteria and smells unpleasant!

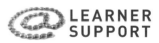

LEARNER SUPPORT

Shampooing crossword

Rinsing and finishing off

After you have completed the shampoo(s), remove all traces of lather and residual shampoo from the hair and scalp. If any residue remains, it could cause irritation and prevent any following services from being completed satisfactorily. Check that the hair is rinsed well by running your fingers through the hair as if you were separating it and feeling for a "slight" greasiness. Well-rinsed hair should feel "squeaky clean" and have some form of resistance between your fingers. After checking the hair, carefully remove the excess water by gently squeezing. The hair is now ready for conditioning.

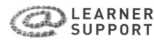

LEARNER SUPPORT

Shampooing wordsearch

EKU statement

GH1 (eku27) how to apply conditioning products to the hair

EKU statement

GH1 (eku29) the importance of detangling the hair from point to root

GH1.3 Apply conditioners to the hair

Science

pH balance
The natural acid mantle of skin and hair has a **pH balance** of 5.5. Conditioners can be used to help rebalance the pH levels of hair to the natural slightly acidic value of hair and skin at pH5.5, particularly after chemical processes such as perming and colouring.

EKU statement

GH1 (eku18) different types of conditioning products and their effects

@ TUTOR SUPPORT

Task 5.8 Situations when not to use conditioner chart

Following the stylist's instructions

Before you apply a conditioner

You must always ask the stylist before applying conditioner to the client's hair to ensure that any following services are not affected. Conditioner will put a thin laminating layer on the outside of the hair, and although this improves handling, it can be a barrier for some other chemical processes. For example, if you have shampooed in preparation for perming, a conditioner could prevent even penetration by the lotion to the hair and this could affect the overall perm result.

Using the appropriate technique

One of the main roles for hairdressers is to improve and maintain the condition of our clients' hair. If the cuticle surface of the client's hair is roughened or damaged, the appearance will be dull. Clients want their hair to shine; therefore we have to improve the surface by "filling in" the missing or damaged areas of cuticle in order to make it as smooth as possible. We do this with help from conditioners. Conditioners make the hair easier to manage, easier to comb and easier to brush.

What are the benefits of using conditioners?

Professional products are formulated to protect and improve a range of different hair types and disorders. The main benefits of using conditioners are that they will:

- smooth the cuticle edges
- improve the handling and combing when the hair is both wet and dry
- temporarily repair and fill damaged sites along the hair shaft or missing areas of the cuticle or cortex

- provide shine, lustre and sheen
- create flexibility and movement by locking in moisture
- balance the pH value of the hair to a slightly acid 5.5.

Types of conditioner

- There are 2 types of conditioner: surface conditioners and treatment conditioners.

Surface conditioners These conditioners work on the surface of the hair. Their main purpose is to coat the cuticle layer of the hair and improve the handling, by making it easier to comb through; and the look and feel, by adding shine and moisture.

Some conditioning rinses are used after perms and chemical straighteners as anti-oxidants (**anti-oxidant conditioners**) to stop any further oxidation, or to balance pH (**pH balance** conditioners).

Treatment conditioners These conditioners penetrate deeper into the hair. Their main purpose is to enter the **cortex,** through the damaged areas of **cuticle** and to fill the air spaces caused by chemical or thermal damage; and replenish the moisture levels within the hair to make it flexible, elastic and add shine and improve handling.

EKU *statement*

GH1 (eku14) the direction in which the hair cuticle lies and its importance when disentangling wet hair

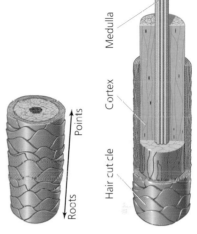

These images show a cross-section through hair showing the different parts. Notice that the "free" edges of cuticle point towards the ends of the hair and not the roots.

Activity

To complete this activity, copy the table below into your portfolio and then for each conditioner that your salon uses at the basin, complete the missing information. Use as many rows as you need.

Conditioning product	Who is the manufacturer?	What hair type is it for?	What does the product do?

Step by step: conditioning

Each conditioning treatment is specific to the task in hand. It is therefore extremely important to follow the manufacturer's instructions so that the product can do its job. Some require heat assisted from a hood dryer or a steamer for deeper penetration into more damaged types of hair. The following sequence provides guidelines for applying a general surface conditioner.

Step 1 After shampooing, squeeze out excess moisture from the hair.

Step 2 Apply a small amount of conditioner into the palm of the hand and gently rub your hands together, applying the conditioner evenly to a wider surface area.

Step 3 On longer hair, apply the conditioner to mid-lengths and ends first, working through the hair with the fingers, separating the lengths.

Step 4 On short hair, evenly apply the conditioner to all of the hair.

Step 5 Then start the petrissage movements over the scalp from the frontal area, over the top and down through to the nape. Repeat this circular process several times.

Step 6 On longer hair that is in poorer condition, you may need to comb the conditioner through whilst still at the basin. Using a wide-toothed conditioning comb, start disentangling the hair, working at the points of the hair first, and then gradually working a little further up the hair, until the hair can be combed easily from roots to ends.

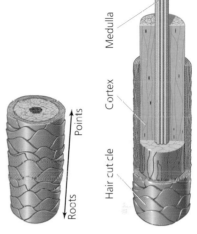

Lee Moran @ Sanrizz

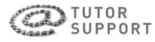

TUTOR SUPPORT

Task 5.9 Investigate conditioners used in the salon

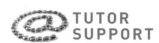

TUTOR SUPPORT

Task 5.10 Different uses for conditioning chart

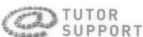
TUTOR SUPPORT

Task 5.11 Discuss what could go wrong when shampooing and conditioning?

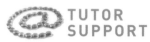
TUTOR SUPPORT

Short answer tests

Rinsing and finishing off

Step 7 Finally rinse all traces of conditioner away from the hair and lightly squeeze out the excess water. If the entire product is not rinsed from the hair; it may act as a barrier to any following processes.

Step 8 Place the towel around the hair, secure into place and move the client to a styling section.

Step 9 Place another fresh towel around the client's shoulders and remove the damp one squeezing out the excess moisture from the lengths.

Step 10 Disentangle the hair with a wide-toothed comb until all tangles are free from the hair remembering to comb from the roots to the points in the direction of the cuticle.

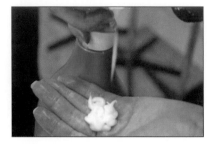
Step 1–4 using the dispenser to meter the correct amount of conditioner

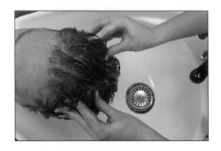
Step 5 an even and balanced conditioning massage

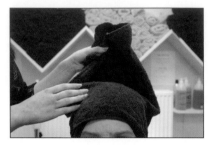
Step 8–10 securing a towel around the head before leaving the basin

Remember

Health and safety

● Raising the client too quickly from the basin can be dangerous. It may make some people feel dizzy when they try to stand up. If they have had any neck problems, it could cause injury.

● Make sure that you do not apply too much pressure on the back of the neck or "joggle" the client's head around by wrongly applying uneven pressure on either side.

● Always test the water temperature on the back of your hands before transferring the flow to the client's head. Look out for changes and fluctuations in water temperatures and pressures.

Activity

Self assessment for shampooing and conditioning

1 I know what the effleurage movement is and when to use this massage technique?
yes ☐   no ☐

2 I know what the rotary movement is and when to use this massage technique?
yes ☐   no ☐

3 I know what the friction movement is and when to use this massage technique?
yes ☐   no ☐

4 I know what the petrissage movement is and when to use this massage technique?
yes ☐   no ☐

5 I know why and how to de-tangle client's hair properly?
yes ☐   no ☐

6 I know how to dispense the right amount of sampoo product for a client?
yes ☐   no ☐

7 I know how to dispense the right amount of conditioning product for a client?
yes ☐   no ☐

8 I can regulate the water pressure and temperature properly?
yes ☐   no ☐

Supervisor's signature: ....   **Date:** ....

Checkerboard

| I know how to prepare the client correctly for shampooing and conditioning treatments ☐ | I know how to check the stock levels of backwash products and how to refill them ☐ | I can always shampoo and condition any client's hair within 5 minutes ☐ |

I know the different massage techniques and when they are used ☐

I know how contact dermatitis can occur and how it can be avoided ☐

I understand the implications of backwash product in relation to personal health and safety ☐

I always make sure that the client is comfortable throughout the process of shampooing and conditioning hair ☐

I always follow the stylist's instructions regarding the use of products and equipment ☐

I understand the implications of poor posture, cleaning and personal hygiene ☐

I know how to shampoo and condition a wide range of hair lengths correctly ☐

I always follow the manufacturer's instructions ☐

I know what surface conditioning is, the application techniques and the benefits to the client's hair ☐

I know how much product to use and how to minimise waste ☐

Revision questions

Q1   Fill in the blank: Shampooing cleans hair by _____ dirt, skin scale and product build up.

Q2   Conditioning treatments raise the hair cuticle. True or false?

Q3   By which of the following methods do conditioners work on the hair? (You may choose more than one answer.)

1	attraction	4	absorption
2	repulsion	5	friction
3	erosion	6	propulsion

Q4   Shampoos contain bleach. True or false?

Q5   The detergent in shampoo lifts grease off hair by suspending it in water. What is this called? (Choose one answer.)

A	hydrophobic	C	emulsion
B	hydrophilic	D	erosion

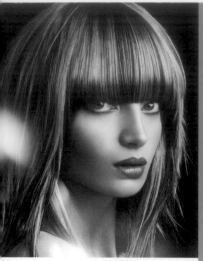

Chapter**six**
Blow dry hair

RAE PALMER FOR SCHWARZKOPF,
PHOTOGRAPHY
ANDREW O'TOOLE **GH2**

GH2.1

GH2.2

**CREDIT VALUE
FOR UNIT GH2**
4 Credits

Unit title

GH2 Blow dry hair

This is an **optional** unit for
Level 1. It is made up of 2
main outcomes.

Main outcomes

GH2 (eku1) Maintain effective and safe methods of
working when drying hair

GH2 (eku2) Blow dry hair

Unit GH2: quick overview

What do I need to do for GH2.1?

You need to **prepare for blow drying** by:

● Correctly protect and position clients and yourself

● keeping the work area clean and safe to use at all times

● maintaining personal hygiene standards

● using tools and resources safely

● completing the service efficiently

What do I need to do for GH2.2?

You need to **blow dry hair** by:

● following the stylist's instructions

● applying the products correctly

● maintaining the client's comfort

● using brushes to style hair professionally

What things do I need to cover?

You will be:

● using flat and round brushes

● working on shorter and longer hair lengths

● creating volume, adding movement and straightening hair

What things do I need to know?

You need to **know and understand**:

- your salon's way of preparing and protecting the clients
- your salon's expectations in standards of service
- how to maintain the work area
- how to work safely and hygienically at all times
- how to maintain and prepare blow drying tools
- what the stylist wants you to do
- why you should check the client's comfort throughout
- the basic structure of hair and how heat and humidity affects the hair
- how to use the tools to create different blow dried effects
- the variety of styling products available and how they are used

Introduction

In this chapter, you will be learning one of the most useful and essential everyday styling techniques and carrying it out on the clients.

This is it – your chance to do what the stylists do!

Blow drying has been the most popular styling technique for several decades. Its popularity has grown in the belief that professional, final effects can be achieved quickly and easily, and that hair maintenance is low. This chapter covers all the things associated with the service: you will be learning how to style hair with different types of brushes and how products can be used to help create the effects. It is simple when you know how.

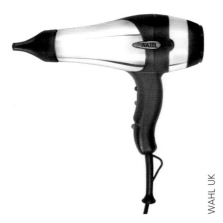

WAHL UK

The hair dryer: your essential tool in the salon

Keywords

Alpha keratin
the state the hair is in before stretching and setting into a new shape

Beta keratin
the state the hair is in after it has been stretched and set into a new shape

Cortex
the inner part of the hair where most chemical processes take place

Cuticle
the outer protective layer of the hair resembling overlapping tiles on a roof

Humidity
the levels of moisture in the air

Medulla
the central part of the hair that is only found in coarser hair types

GH2.1 Maintain effective and safe methods of working when drying hair

EKU statement

GH2 (eku1) your salon's requirements for client preparation

GH2 (eku5) the range of protective clothing that should be available for clients

GH2 (eku7) the safety considerations which must be taken into account when blow drying hair

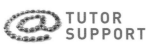

TUTOR SUPPORT

Task 6.1 List: Health and safety

EKU statement

GH2 (eku6) how the position of your client and yourself can affect the desired outcome and reduce fatigue and the risk of injury

EKU statement

GH2 (eku3) your salon's requirements for the disposal of waste

GH2 (eku9) why it is important to keep your work area clean and tidy

Remember

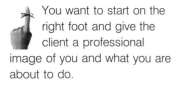

You want to start on the right foot and give the client a professional image of you and what you are about to do.

Correctly protect and position clients and yourself

Blow drying is a finishing service, like setting or finger drying, so it will always follow some other services, even if only shampooing. That means that the client will arrive at the styling unit with wet hair. Their clothes must be protected from accidental spills with a clean, freshly laundered gown.

The first thing you need to do is make sure that, if the towel is taken away, the client's hair will not drip. This is not a safety issue, but a feature of good customer care and attention to detail, especially if the client has long hair. Remove excess moisture by gently squeezing the hair in the towel or by light rubbing. Put the damp towel aside and put a clean, dry, fresh towel around the shoulders and secure it with a clip. Take a wide-tooth comb and, working through the ends of the hair first, carefully start to detangle the client's hair. Work at small areas of hair starting at the nape and then work around the head until all of the hair has been combed and is free of knots.

Work position

Salon chairs are designed with comfort and safety in mind; your client's back should be flat against the back of the chair and the chair at a comfortable height for you to work. You need to get to all parts of the head without having to over-reach or stretch, so adjust the chair's height to suit your height and the comfort of the client. Don't be afraid to ask the client to sit up. If the client slouches, their head and neck will be at an angle that makes styling almost impossible; also, their posture will quickly cause them back pain and possible injury.

Your posture

As a stylist or barber, your standing position is equally important to avoid injury. Stand close enough to the styling chair so that you stand upright when either working from:

- a **side of the chair position** – so as to not raise your arms above shoulder height at any time during the service to avoid pain and muscle fatigue
- the **back of the chair position** – the mirror in front of you, with a clear view of the client's head to see the shape of their hair as you are styling.

Keeping the work area clean and safe to use at all times

Prepare any equipment or styling products that you need beforehand. If you use a trolley as a workstation, have your trolley prepared with all the materials you will need. Remove all items and waste from the shelves before any client sits at the styling unit, including:

- combs, brushes and sectioning clips
- magazines, papers etc.
- any previously used materials
- mugs, cups and saucers
- styling and finishing products.

The work space should be tidy; working surfaces should be cleaned with a disinfecting spray, and the mirror polished. The whole work area should be hygienic and give the client a positive and professional image.

For more information on salon cleaning and general salon hygiene, see Chapter 4, Prepare for hair services and maintain work areas.

Maintaining personal hygiene standards

All the materials that come into contact with the client's skin and hair must be clean and hygienic. Similarly, your own personal standards of health and hygiene should not present any risk to client. This will prevent the risk of cross-infection and helps to maintain a healthy safe environment. For more information on preventing infection, and personal health and hygiene, see Chapter 1, Make sure your own actions reduce risks to health and safety, pages 4–22.

Activity

Different salons have different ways of doing things. Find out what your salon's policy is in respect to:

1 preparing the client prior to styling

2 preparing tools and equipment ready for use

3 the use of styling products within the salon

4 retail products and how they are brought up in conversation with the client.

Using tools and resources safely

All the tools that you use must be hygienic and safe for use. They must be cleaned and sterilised before they can be used on the client. You can review the section covering sterilisation and tool maintenance in Chapter 4, Prepare for hair services and maintain work areas, page 56.

With the client sitting ready at the styling unit, you need to be ready with the:

- flat and round brushes that you will be using in the UV cabinet
- combs, sectioning clips, etc., which will need to be rinsed after removing from the Barbicide™
- blow dryer's lead unravelled, straightened and plugged in, ready to use.

Brushes

Different brushes do different jobs and if you use the wrong type of brush it has a detrimental effect on the finished look. The length of the hair and the client's style dictates the type of brush you need to use. There are two main types of brushes: round and flat – note how they are used and maintained.

EKU statement

GH2 (eku10) why it is important to clean, disinfect and sterilise tools

GH2 (eku11) the difference between disinfection and sterilisation

GH2 (eku12) methods of cleaning, disinfecting and/or sterilisation used in salons

GH2 (eku13) methods of working safely and hygienically and which minimise the risk of cross-infection and cross-infestation

EKU statement

GH2 (eku8) why it is important to avoid cross-infection and infestation

GH2 (eku15) the importance of personal hygiene

Remember

 Always follow the stylist's instructions for completing the hairstyle. Don't just do what you feel will be right – it might be wrong!

EKU statement

GH2 (eku14) the correct use and maintenance of blow drying tools

EKU statement

GH2 (eku22) the range of flat and round brushes available for blow drying

Remember

Avoid cross-infection and cross-infestation: always use cleaned and sterilised brushes on the clients.

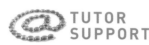
TUTOR SUPPORT

Task 6.2 Brushes used

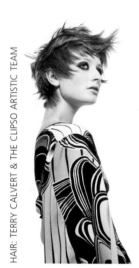

HAIR: TERRY CALVERT & THE CLIPSO ARTISTIC TEAM

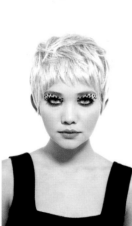

HAIR: TERRY CALVERT & THE CLIPSO ARTISTIC TEAM

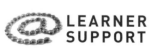
LEARNER SUPPORT

Hot cross bun sectioning for one length cut video

Round & Flat Brushes

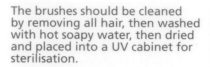

Bristles

The brushes should be cleaned by removing all hair, then washed with hot soapy water, then dried and placed into a UV cabinet for sterilisation.

Remember to turn after 20 mins to do both sides.

The bristles should be straight without heat damage. Any damaged brushes should not be used as they can harbour germs.

Handle

A good, professional brush will either have a rubber handle or shaped grip. This makes it easier to hold and more stable when you are turning and shaping the hair.

DENMAN

DENMAN

Round and flat brushes – note how they are used and maintained

Styling tools and their applications

Denman Classic Styling brush This is the flat brush shown in the picture.

- **Uses**: detangling hair (before shampooing, styling and blow drying straight hair of any length).
- **Description**: a parallel, flat brush with removable plastic cushioned bristles. Available in small (5 rows), medium (7 rows), and large (9 rows) of bristles. The more rows of teeth, the wider the surface area of the styling brush.
- **Technique**: Blow drying is achieved by placing the leading edge of the bristles against the mesh of hair then turning the brush to engage the hair across the whole width. The brush is used from roots to points, with the dryer blowing across the cushioned surface.
- **Cleaning and maintenance**: Denman brushes can be dismantled by removing the rubber cushioned head from the brush handle and the bristle rows can be removed and washed in hot soapy water, then dried and replaced. Rows of bristles can be replaced if damaged or overheated.

Vented brush

- **Uses**: blow drying straight short and mid-length hair.
- **Description**: a parallel, flat brush with a double row of rigid plastic bristles (short and long) affixed to a brush head that is not solid. Allows air to pass between the bristles.
- **Technique**: blow drying is achieved by placing the leading edge of the bristles against the mesh of hair then turning the brush to engage the hair across the whole width. The brush is used from roots to points with the dryer blowing across the cushioned surface.

- **Cleaning and maintenance**: vented brushes can be cleaned by raking out any loose or tangled hair from the bristles, then washing in hot soapy water. The brush is then dried before use.

Paddle brush

- **Uses**: general brushing, detangling hair and pre-dressing hair.
- **Description**: a flat brush with a wide head, usually with a cushioned head and wider teeth than a Denman. Sometimes the bristles are natural in composition, but generally they are plastic.
- **Technique**: paddle brushes are generally too wide to use for blow drying, although sections can be dried by placing sections of hair upon the brush and drying by drawn down from the roots to the points of the hair.
- **Cleaning and maintenance**: paddle brushes can be cleaned by raking out any loose or tangled hair from the bristles, then washing in hot soapy water. The brush is then dried before use.

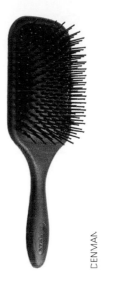

DENMAN

Round brush This is the round brush shown in the picture.

- **Uses**: blow drying with volume, lift, wave and curl on shorter or longer length hair.
- **Description**: round, also known as radial, brushes are completely round and come in a wide variety of sizes. The bristles are usually made of plastic, although pure bristle brushes are still available. The inner body of radial brushes are often made of metal, allowing the brush to heat up. This improves the drying speeds of the underneath hair within a section.
- **Technique**: blow drying volume and movement is achieved by placing meshes of damp hair around the brush and drying the hair in position from both sides. When dry, the curl or movement can be fixed or set into position by applying a cool shot to increase the durability of the set.
- **Cleaning and maintenance**: radial brushes can be cleaned by raking out any loose or tangled hair from the bristles, then washing in hot soapy water. The brush is then dried before use.

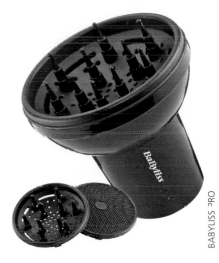

BABYLISS PRO

Diffuser This is not a brush. It is a piece of equipment used to finger-dry the hair.

- **Uses**: scrunch-drying and finger-drying hair to optimise the natural or permed movement within the hair.
- **Description**: a diffuser is an attachment for a blow dryer that suppresses the blast of hot air and turns it into a multidirectional diffused heat.
- **Technique**: the hair is styled with the fingers by either pressing into the cupped diffuser to dry or by working through the hair with the fingers until the hair is dried with the required amount of texture or definition.
- **Cleaning and maintenance**: diffusers are cleaned by spraying with an antibacterial spray then wiped with paper towels.

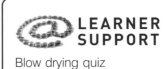 **LEARNER SUPPORT**

Blow drying quiz

Blow dryers

A good professional blow dryer should have the following features:

- at least two speeds
- at least two heat settings
- a variety of detachable shaped nozzles to channel the heat onto the brush or comb
- a lead long enough so that it doesn't tangle around the chair or client

Remember

Always check the condition of the lead and plug before attempting to plug the dryer into the mains socket. If it looks damaged or the cable is broken, tell your supervisor immediately.

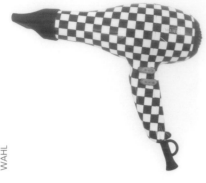

WAHL

A good professional blow dryer

EKU *statement*

GH2 (eku2) your salon's expected service times for basic blow drying services

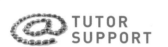

TUTOR SUPPORT

Discussion 6.1: Time requirements

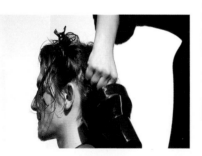

Finger-drying using a diffuser

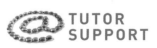

TUTOR SUPPORT

Short answer tests

- it should be powerful enough to dry damp hair quickly (1200w–1500w)
- it should have a cool shot button to enable hot hair to be fixed (set) into shape around a brush
- it should not be too long, so that it is balanced in the hand and can be held away from the client's hair during drying
- it should be light enough so that it can be manipulated easily and used for long periods without fatigue
- it should be quiet enough when in use to allow natural conversation with the client.

Completing the service efficiently

However much fun doing a blow dry may seem, remember to keep to the allotted time:

- do not make the client late, as they may have other plans that day
- do not make the stylist run late – they may need to alter your blow dry afterwards and have other waiting clients
- remain professional – if you are given responsibility, it must be up to standard.

The following table provides a guideline for how long each type of blow-dried style will take:

Hair length	Style	Brush	Time
short	straight	Denman or vented	20 mins
mid-length, bob	straight	Denman or vented	25 mins
long, one length	straight	large round	35 mins
short	volume and lift or curly	small round	25 mins
mid-length, layered	movement and texture	medium round	30 mins
long, layered	movement and texture	large round and medium round	40 mins
medium, layered	curly	small round	35 mins
long, layered	curly	medium round and small round	45 mins

Make sure that you always:

✔	Wash your hands before attending to any clients
✔	Wear a minimum of jewellery, so that doesn't dangle or tangle in the client's hair
✔	Wear comfortable (flatter and not open-toed) footwear when on the salon floor
✔	Be aware of bad breath use breath fresheners if you do have a problem
✔	Take a shower daily before going to work
✔	Make sure your work-wear is clean and fresh every day
✔	Think how you want to be seen by others – you are an advertisement for the service you offer, so make sure that your hair is clean and styled
✔	Minimise the risk of cross-infection to your colleagues and clients

Science

The effects of humidity on the hair

Blow drying produces a temporary change in the hair's structure as it is dried and reformed into its new shape. This is the **beta keratin** state, the state the hair is in after it has been stretched and set into a new shape. This newly created shape or "set" effect is soon lost if and when moisture is absorbed or introduced to the hair. When this happens, the hair reverts back to its original **alpha keratin** state.

You have probably discovered this effect of humidity yourself. If, after you have done your hair, you take a bath in a steamy bathroom, what happens to the hairstyle? It collapses! Moisture is all around us in the air and, in more extremes of **humidity** it is seen as mist and fog. To help prevent a hairstyle from collapsing, a wide variety of styling products are available that repel or withstand the moisture and to help hair stay in shape longer.

EKU *statement*

GH2 (eku19) the effects of humidity on hair

EKU *statement*

GH2 (eku4) your salon's image and expected standards of service

GH2 (eku16) the importance of checking you have understood the instructions given by the stylist

Science

The signs of hair in good and poor condition

Hair in **good condition** has a smooth, flat **cuticle layer**, tightly closed along the hair shaft – with free edges pointing towards the ends of the hair. Hair in **poor condition** has a raised cuticle; the edges are not flat and feel roughened. This can expose the **cortex below**, making the hair very dry and damaged. See Chapter 5, Shampoo and condition hair, for images of cross-sections through hair and for more information about conditioning.

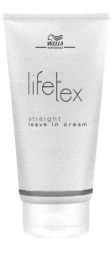

WELLA

Styling products help hair stay in shape by repelling moisture

Following the stylist's instructions

Although you are styling the client's hair, the stylist is ultimately responsible for what you do; therefore, you must follow their instructions and wishes throughout the blow dry. Use only the tools and sequence as they instruct you to. For instance, if they have specifically said that they wanted the back of the client's one length bob sectioned off, and the underneath dried first, then that is where you must start. The stylist will provide you with the instructions required for a satisfactory result in the time available. Any deviation from their instructions will probably cause you to go wrong and possibly leave you with an unhappy client.

If you start struggling, ask the stylist for help. You may find that the client tries to be helpful and may say "I always dry the fringe and the sides first". You should then say politely "I'll ask Steve if that's OK with him".

When you finish the style the client may want or need some finishing products like wax, defining crème, moulding clay or hairspray. Don't apply these products unless you have been told to; leave it to your stylist. A client may often try to help by saying "I always use plenty of gel". But with all due respect to them; you may find yourself in hot water if you don't listen to the expressed wishes of the senior stylist – for example, you may put too much on and the hair will have to be re-shampooed and started all over again!

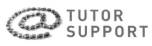

TUTOR SUPPORT

Task 6.3 Structure of the hair

Remember

If the hair is long, you will need to work from the points, through the lengths, back up towards the roots because the ends will always be wetter than the root area.

Activity

Draw a diagram to show the basic structure of the hair. On the diagram show the positions of the **cuticle**, the **cortex** and **medulla**, and indicate which are the root end of the hair and the points of the hair. Now answer the following questions in your portfolio:

1 What are alpha and beta keratin?
2 What does the cuticle layer look like?
3 What are the indicators of hair in good condition?
4 What are the indicators of hair in poor condition?

5 What effect does humidity have on a finished hair style?
6 What is another name for a round brush?
7 Give two examples of flat brushes.

EKU *statement*

GH2 (eku23) the types and purposes of blow drying products

Applying the products correctly

Always try to minimise waste – use care and control when you dispense the products and only use as much as you need; remember, the towels don't need excess styling products, it's just throwing money away.

Applying styling products

Always use styling products sparingly. The following images show how much mousse should be applied to short- to medium-length hair:

- it will either be thrown away or rubbed off into a towel
- it could irritate the client's scalp – excess product could overload the scalp area.

Remember

 Do not overload the hair. This will make the hair unpleasantly hard (unless the style/client requires it). You may have to re-shampoo and start over.

Remember

Use the products sparingly. You can always add more as you need it. Don't apply too much at first.

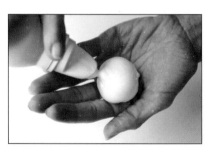

Step 1 Standard styling mousse to be applied to the mid-lengths and ends.

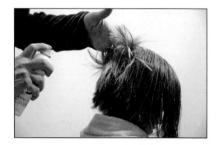

Step 2 Root/volumising mousse being applied to root area by separating the hair and spraying at different points where volume is required.

Applying finishing products

Hairspray   Hairspray fixes hair into shape. Always hold the can upright and at least 30 cm away from the hair. Make sure that the pin-hole in the nozzle faces the client's hair and lightly mist for a few seconds.

Moulding/defining crème   Moulding/defining crème adds texture and hold. It is ideal for adding texture to layered hairstyles. Take a small amount of product onto the end of your index finger. Transfer this to your inner fingers on both hands evenly and then work into the outer layers to create the textured effect. Add more to create the desired effect.

Serum   Serum provides control and shine, and smoothes down frizzies. This product is available as light hair oils or moisturising control crèmes. Apply a couple of drops to the fingers and work together between the fingers on both hands. Apply carefully and evenly throughout the lengths to improve the look and feel of the hair.

Always hold the hairspray can at least 30 cm from the hair

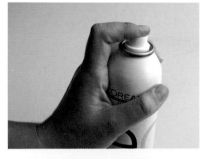

Take a small amount of moulding crème onto the end of your index finger

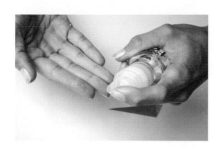

A small amount of serum, a light hair oil

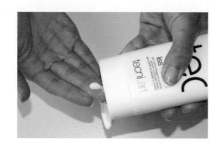

Moisturising control crème

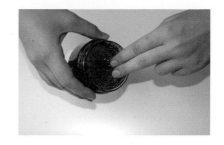

Gel provide a strong, wet look

Gel Gel provides a strong, wet look hold in any hair type. It is ideal for adding strong spiky texture to layered hairstyles. To use, take a small amount of product onto the ends of your fingers. Transfer this to your fingers on both hands evenly and then work into the outer layers to create the textural effect. Add more to create the sculpted effect.

Wax Wax provides strong, medium or soft hold in any textured hairstyle. Take a small amount of product onto the end of your index finger. Transfer this to your fingertips on both hands evenly and then work into the outer hair. Add more to create the textured effect.

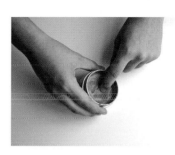

Wax provides strong, medium or soft hold in any textured hairstyle

Product	What is it for?	How is it applied?	When do you use it?
styling mousse	a general styling aid for adding volume and providing hold	blob the size of a small orange evenly to the lengths	on dampened hair before sectioning and drying
root lift mousse	a special mousse that has a directional nozzle, allowing you to apply foam at or near to the roots	lift and separate sections of dampened hair so that the root area is exposed; hold the can so that the nozzle aims the foam near the root	on hair that needs body but doesn't require setting hold at the mid-lengths and points
styling gel/glaze	a wet look, firm hold finish on shorter hair styles	small "pea sized" amount from the finger tips all over evenly (you can always add more if necessary)	not easy to blow dry, can be used in finger drying and scrunch dry techniques
moulding clay	a dual purpose product for styling or finishing that bonds the hair with firm hold	on damp hair: a small "pea sized" amount from the finger tips all over evenly; on dry hair; with finger tips to the points of the hair for texture and definition	a firm textural bond on most lengths of hair
defining crème	a finishing product that provides control on unruly hair	on dry hair: small "droplet" amounts a little at a time with finger tips	throughout the lengths of the hair for smooth control and conditioning
defining wax	a slightly greasy finishing product that provides textural effects to short to longer hair	on dry hair: apply small "pea sized" amounts a little at a time with finger tips	throughout the ends of the hair for style definition and/or textural effects
serum	a slightly oily finishing product that provides improved handling and shine	on dry hair: small droplet amounts a little at a time with finger tips	throughout the lengths of the hair for smooth control and better conditioning

Product	What is it for?	How is it applied?	When do you use it?
hairspray	a finishing product in a variety of holds/strengths, pump or aerosol spray	mist hair from about 30–40 cm away from the hair for a "fixed" hold on dry hair	final fixative, overall sealer or a scrunching, textural finish
dry wax	a non-greasy finishing product that provides textural effects on short to longer hair	on dry hair: small "pea sized" amounts a little at a time with finger tips	used throughout the ends of the hair for style definition and/or textural effects

Remember

The way that you approach the work will say a lot about your levels of ability to the client. Be confident, be careful – but above all, be professional!

Note: always follow the manufacturer's instructions when handling styling and finishing products. See Chapter 1, Make sure your own actions reduce risks to health and safety, and Appendix 1, COSHH Regulations.

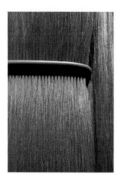

Use serum for smooth control and better conditioning

Activity

Product knowledge

For each of the products listed below, find out which sorts of hair styles they are most appropriate for. Try to find examples of these in style magazines or from websites on the internet and put these and your answers in you portfolio.

Product	Suitable styles and lengths
soft wax	
gel	
moulding clay	
serum	
mousse	
hard wax	

Remember

Never try to dry saturated hair; you need to work upon hair that is damp rather than wet, so dry off the hair in the areas that need it first. You can always re-moisten the hair if it becomes too dry.

EKU *statement*

GH2 (eku17) the importance of checking client comfort throughout the drying process

Maintaining the client's comfort

Always check with the client to see that they are comfortable throughout the service. Mind how you use the dryer and direct the heat over the surface of the brush when blow drying. If the blast of heat and air deflects off the edge that is nearest the client's scalp, you will burn them. They will be really annoyed, you will look foolish, and the professional bond of respect will be lost!

Using brushes to style hair professionally

These images show the correct position of the dryer in relation to both the brush and the direction of the heat.

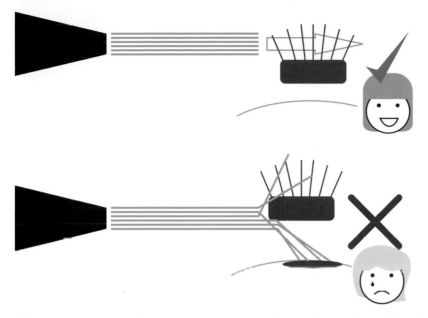

EKU *statement*

GH2 (eku21) how the incorrect application of heat can affect the hair and scalp

GH2 (eku7) the safety considerations which must be taken into account when blow drying hair

GH2 (eku24) why and how to use flat and round brushes to create volume, movement and to straighten hair

This is the correct angle to hold a brush in relation to the position of the client's head. The heat from a wrongly positioned brush will burn the client within 2 or 3 seconds, regardless of which heat setting and which speed you are using.

Drying the hair – roots to points

You should only work on small sections, no larger that the surface area of the brush you are using. If the sections are too large, you will not be able to dry each mesh of hair properly. This will affect the durability of the finished look. Be careful not to over-heat any sections of the hair while you are drying. The effects are long term and will damage the hair.

Start the blow dry at the lower back. Section out of the way any surplus hair and secure it with a clip. Then, taking your dryer in one hand, offer the dryer across to the section to check the angle of the nozzle. The air should be parallel to the angle of the hair. Take your brush in the other hand and introduce the bristles to the hair near the root area. Pick up and turn the brush so that the hair is caught across the bristles. Turn on the dryer and, now aiming across the brush, follow the brush downwards with the dryer, holding it about 10–15 cm away.

Focusing the jet stream

The hair can only dry if the blast from the dryer is working over the surface of it. So bearing this in mind, carefully aim the flat, jet stream of heated air across the surface of the brush, shielding the heat from the back (scalp side) side of the brush. As you move the brush down, move the dryer down so that it mirrors the position of the brush at always the same distance away. Blow drying from root to point ensures that the cuticle lays flat therefore reducing fly-away frizz and smoothing the overall result.

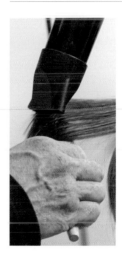

See how the brush is held in relation to the blow dryer

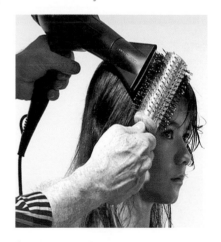

See how the brush is held in relation to the client's head

Remember

Water moisture will naturally fall and run down the hair shaft with gravity, so starting near the root area will always quicken the drying process. After a couple of passes through the hair, the section will be dry.

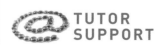
TUTOR SUPPORT

Task 6.4 Investigate styling products

If you are using a round, radial brush you will find that you need to take a section and wind the hair around the brush. Again, focus the jet stream over the curved surfaces of the brush, but this time from both sides. This will enable the hair to dry around the brush, forming part of the wave. Then after drying and while still warm, use a cool shot from the dryer (or use "blast only" without heat settings) to "freeze" the wave into place. (This fixes the style with more durability, like in setting – when rollers are allowed to cool down before removal and final brushing and dressing out.) If you do not allow the meshes of hair to cool, the result will be less firm and will not last as long. Finally, with the section dry, you can take down another mesh, ready for drying into position.

Working with tensioned hair

You have to maintain an even tension on the meshes of hair throughout the blow drying service. This ensures that the hair will dry with a smooth, sleek effect without frizzies or crimped areas. If you do create a kinked, uneven result, you can lightly spray down with water and start again. Look out for the hair in the sectioning clips waiting to be dried too. If the hair has a natural tendency to wave or curl, it might disfigure it before you can style it. Again, lightly mist it down with water and start over.

Step-by-step: blow drying short hair

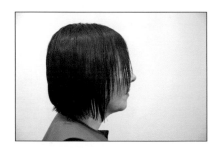

Step 1 After shampooing and conditioning, detangle the hair and position the client's parting.

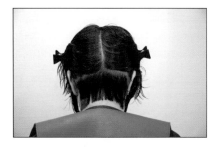

Step 2 The blow dry is started at the back. Section off the hair horizontally and neatly in the true professional way.

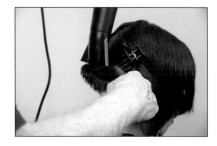

Step 3 Start by placing the hair around the brush evenly – hold the dryer above the section as shown.

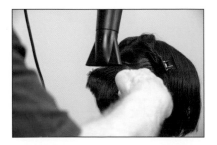

Step 4 Make sure that the hot jet of air glances off the brush away from the client's head.

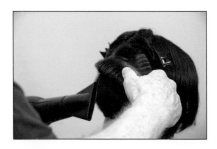

Step 5 You can carefully dry the ends by turning the dryer around – this provides even, smooth lift and volume.

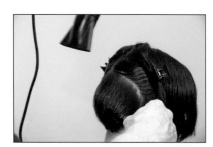

Step 6 Work up the back of the hair style by taking a new section down to work with.

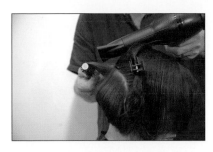

Step 7 This view clearly shows the correct drying angle for drying each section – never hold the heat on the hair for too long.

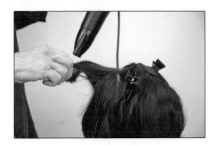

Step 8 Keep the brush moving with a circular movement in your hand as you dry the hair and keeping an even tension.

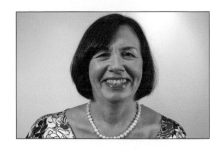

Step 9 Continue with the same technique until all of the hair is finished.

Step-by-step: Blow drying long hair

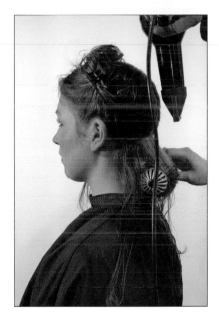

Step 1 Divide the hair at the back so that the nape can be blow dried first.

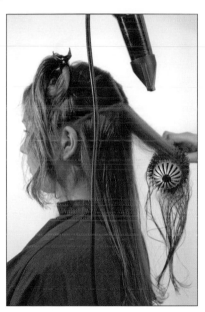

Step 2 Work up the back, finishing and drying each section before moving on to the next.

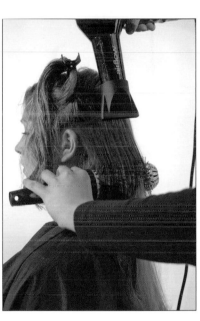

Step 3 Continue up the back, keeping the angle of the dryer parallel with the hair.

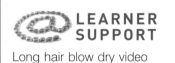

LEARNER SUPPORT

Long hair blow dry video

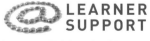

LEARNER SUPPORT

Long radial brush video blowdry

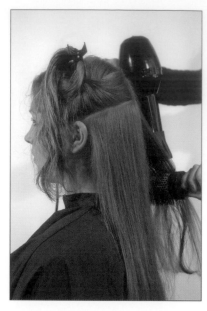

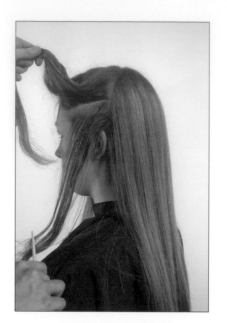

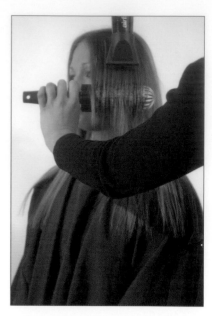

Step 4 Take each section down and dry in the same way.

Step 5 With the back complete, you can start at the lower side, remembering to section the hair out of the way.

Step 6 The finished effect.

Finger drying

Finger drying is a fast and more natural way of drying hair into style. After removing excess moisture from the hair, some mousse can be applied to provide some body and texture to work with. The main idea of finger drying is to use a blow dryer with the fingers in a directional drying process, on generally shorter hair. The fingers provide 2 main benefits for this technique:

- they allow a style to be moulded on hair that would normally be too short to dry with brushes
- they can be used to style longer hair into cascades of curly movement, either on natural or permed hair.

Remember

 When finger drying hair:

always work with damp and not saturated hair – rough-dry if necessary

- work on small areas/ sections of hair
- try to dry the hair in the direction of roots to points – it will dry more quickly and keep the cuticle layer smoother, making it look healthier and shinier
- avoid burning the scalp – angle your dryer away from the head
- move the position of your client's head in order to get around, and cover all areas of the head
- use both hands to dry the hair – so swap the dryer around, as this allows you to work on both sides of the head effectively.

Activity
Product knowledge

Copy the table below into your portfolio. Then complete the missing information to show how and when the products are applied.

Product	How is it applied?	When is it applied?
mousse		
root mousse		
styling gel		
serum		
defining crème		
hair wax		

Blow dry styling dos and don'ts

Do	Don't
Do dry the hair well so that it's moist but not wet before starting the blow dry.	**Don't** leave damp towels around the client's shoulders.
Do take small sections that you can control and dry evenly throughout.	**Don't** leave the dryer running whilst you re-section the hair.
Do direct the flow of air away from the client.	**Don't** use the top heat setting unless it's really necessary.
Do adjust the chair height so you can reach the top of the client's head without over-stretching.	**Don't** pass the brushes to the client for them to hold in between sectioning.
Do ask the client to adjust their head position if you need to.	**Don't** try to use the same hand for brush work on both sides of the head.
Do clip out of the way any sections that are not yet being worked on.	**Don't** over-dry the hair, as this will cause permanent damage.

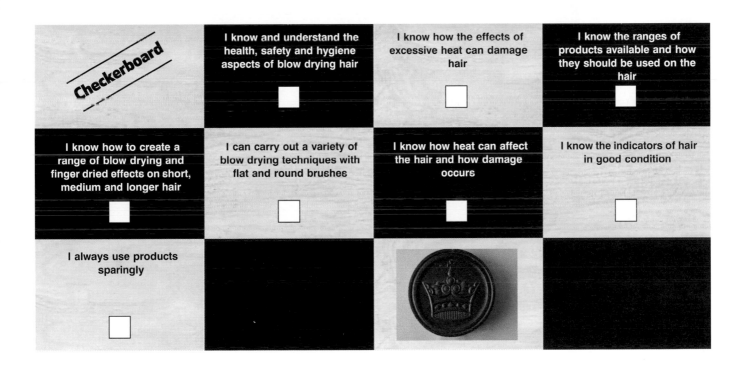

Checkerboard

I know and understand the health, safety and hygiene aspects of blow drying hair ☐

I know how the effects of excessive heat can damage hair ☐

I know the ranges of products available and how they should be used on the hair ☐

I know how to create a range of blow drying and finger dried effects on short, medium and longer hair ☐

I can carry out a variety of blow drying techniques with flat and round brushes ☐

I know how heat can affect the hair and how damage occurs ☐

I know the indicators of hair in good condition ☐

I always use products sparingly ☐

Revision questions

Q1 Fill in the blank: Brushes can be ——— by putting them into a UV cabinet.

Q2 A round brush is also called a radial brush. True or false?

Q3 Which of the following are types of blow drying brushes? (You may choose more than one answer.)

1	flat	**4**	oval
2	square	**5**	round
3	oblong	**6**	triangular

Q4 The bristles of brushes are normally made from plastics. True or false?

Q5 Hair is changed into what state during the process of blow drying? (Choose one answer.)

a	alpha keratin	**c**	permanent set
b	beta keratin	**d**	damaged

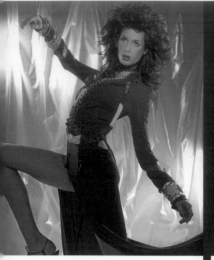

Chapter**seven**
Assist with hair colouring services

HAIR: RICHARD WARD, PHOTOGRAPHY: DANIELE CIPRIANI

GH4

GH4.1

GH4.2

CREDIT VALUE FOR UNIT GH4

4 Credits

Unit title

GH4 Assist with hair colouring services

This is an **optional** unit for Level 1. It is made up of 2 main outcomes.

Main outcomes

GH4 (eku1) Maintain effective and safe methods of working when assisting with colouring services

GH4 (eku2) Remove colouring and lightening products

Unit GH4: quick overview

What do I need to do for GH4.1?

You need to **prepare for removing colours** by:

- learning why hair is different colours
- learning about colouring techniques
- correctly protect and position the client and yourself
- maintaining personal hygiene standards
- keeping the work area clean and safe to use at all times
- identifying when colours need reordering

What do I need to do for GH4.2?

You need to **remove colours** by:

- minimising the risk of hair damage
- keeping the client adequately protected
- applying suitable conditioners
- leaving the client ready for further services

What things do I need to cover?

You will be removing:

- semi-permanent colours
- quasi-permanent colours
- permanent colours
- lightening products

What things do I need to know?

You need to **know and understand**:

- your salon's way of preparing and protecting the clients
- your salon's procedures for the disposal of waste items
- your responsibilities in respect to COSHH
- what contact dermatitis is and how to avoid developing it
- how the Data Protection Act affects client records
- how to clean and prepare the salon's work areas
- how to work safely and hygienically at all times
- the importance of rinsing the hair thoroughly
- how to emulsify a colour during the removal
- why you should follow instructions when removing colouring products
- the types of problems that could occur

Introduction

A colouring service is a complex technical process; it covers a variety of different methods for changing the colour of a client's hair. Most colouring services take a long time.

The result of colouring hair is well worth the wait!

The removal of colours and particularly the multi-coloured effects of highlighting are critical to achieving a successful result – and you play a key role in helping to achieve this. This chapter helps you to understand the differences between colours and lighteners and explains how you can assist the stylists in their work.

EKU *statement*

GH4 (eku1) your salon's requirements for client preparation

GH4 (eku2) your salon's and legal requirements for disposal of waste materials

---

GH4.1 — Maintain effective and safe methods of working when assisting with colouring services

Learning why hair is different colours

Hair comes in a wide range of different colours. Some of these are natural hair (**virgin hair**); others are obviously coloured or look like natural hair, but are coloured. The colours range from blonde and brown to black and grey. These colours are made up from **pigments** within the hair. In natural hair these pigments are produced

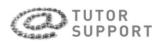

TUTOR SUPPORT

Task 7.1 Explore the concept of hair colour and hair colour services

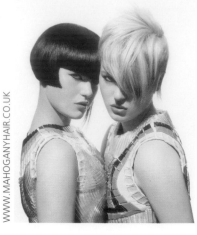

MAHOGANY HAIRDRESSING SALONS & ACADEMT,
WWW.MAHOGANYHAIR.CO.UK

Look at a group of friends – how many colours of hair do you see?

Science

The natural pigments collectively called melanin are made up from **eumelanin** and **pheomelanin**. Eumelanin produces black or brown pigments and pheomelanin gives yellow and red ones. The naturally occurring colours that you see in other people's hair are a mixture of these two pigments. The pigments are so small that it would be the same as looking at grains of sand inside a ball-point pen. Individually the pigments are different in colour, but when seen by the eye they appear to be one colour.

as different forms of **melanin**. In coloured hair, artificial pigments are either added to or replace the natural pigments in the hair.

Types of colour

Semi-permanent colour   Semi-permanent colours are ideal for clients who want colour but don't want it to be permanent. They last up to 6 or 8 shampoos and do not produce any visible re-growth. The hair loses colour on each shampoo, so the effect fades over time. They do not lighten hair; they can only add tones to the existing colour. They contain conditioning agents that add shine and improve style manageability whilst the colour processes.

Quasi-permanent colour   Quasi-permanent colours last longer than semi-permanents but not as long as true permanent colour. They also produce re-growth. They will cover some grey hair and are a popular colour choice for people who colour their hair themselves.

Permanent colour   Permanent colours make up the largest variety of shades and tones. They can cover grey (which is in fact white hair) and modify the natural pigments in the hair to produce a range of natural, fashion and fantasy shades. Hydrogen peroxide is mixed with permanent colour to develop the process; the hair will then retain the colour permanently in the **cortex**. Hair in poor condition, however, will not hold the colour, and colouring could result in patchy areas and colour fading.

Lightener   Lighteners and bleaches contain alkaline chemicals that dissolve the natural pigments in hair. Like permanent colours, lightening products are mixed with hydrogen peroxide. They are used in 3 main forms: high lift colour, powder bleach and cream or oil bleach.

Learning about colouring techniques

Stylists use a variety of classic and contemporary methods to colour their clients' hair. Some of these are easy for you to remove at the basin, whereas others are quite complex. A stylist may colour hair using the following techniques:

- full head colour
- re-growth colour
- "T"-section or full head highlights
- slice or spot colour
- cap highlights.

Semi-permanent colours wash out gradually with each shampoo

Activity

1   What are the colouring services offered at your salon/shop?

2   Does your salon have any particular requirements in the way that colours must be taken off?

3   What materials are used for highlighting services?

List the services available in your salon and the materials that are used to create the effects in your portfolio.

Colour and care

Full head colour This is an application of semi, quasi, permanent colour or lightener to all of the hair, regardless of length. The colour is applied in a certain order so that the client's hair develops to a final, single colour that is even from the root area to the points of the hair. Care must be taken to emulsify the colour so that it releases the colour from the hair, making it easier to shampoo and remove.

Re-growth colour Re-growth colour, also called a retouch, refers to the application of permanent colour or lightener to the hair that has re-grown since the last colour application. It looks like a line or band of natural hair between the scalp and the artificial/synthetic hair colour. Re-growth colours are fairly simple to remove. They are a single colour applied to only part of the head. Like full head colours, they should be emulsified so that the colour removal provides a better result.

"T"-section and full head highlights "T"-section highlights are a popular way of placing highlights along the parting area and down around the sides of the front hairline. "T"-section highlights are usually an in-between option for a client who has a re-growth of natural hair, with highlights still showing within the lengths.

Full head highlights are also a popular technique for creating a multi-toned effect throughout the client's hair. Each meche/foil is carefully positioned so that only the parts requiring colour are processed. The meches keep the colours from merging into the rest of the hair and creating an unwanted and potentially damaging result.

For both, hair may be lightened and/or coloured. Special care needs to be taken during removal so that the (or each individual) colour is carefully removed and is prevented from discolouring other parts of the hair, which creates an unpleasant "muddy" result.

Slice and spot colouring Slice colouring is very similar to highlights, where sections of hair are taken and coloured to produce more striking, dramatic results. Again, the meches/foils keep the colours from merging into the rest of the hair.

Spot colouring is a technique using temporary semi, quasi, permanent colours or lighteners in specific areas in between re-growth or full head colouring. It is often used for colouring white hair that shows in a parting.

The hair may be lightened and/or coloured. Care needs to be taken removing this type of colour so that each individual colour is carefully removed and is prevented from discolouring other parts of the hair.

Cap highlights Cap highlights are a way of producing a uniform highlighted result by pulling sections of hair through a rubber cap and applying colour or lightener. The process is a way of producing a single colour effect. This is a simple and popular option for men's colouring. Providing that the cap is not worn and the holes have not split, the removal of cap highlights is fairly simple. After rinsing, make sure that you lift the flange edge back over the cap all round so that the cap comes away easily without too much tugging.

Correctly protect and position the client and yourself

The preparation for the client at the basin is the same as in shampooing. Please review Chapter 5, Shampoo and condition hair, pages 71–6, for more information.

EKU statement

GH4 (eku18) the manufacturers' instructions for the removal of the specific colouring products and materials in your salon

Remember

 All of these products are chemicals and must be handled in accordance with the manufacturers' instructions. You must wear the correct PPE (non-latex disposable gloves) when handling chemicals.

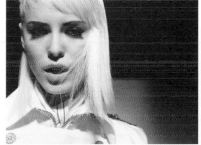

DAMIEN CARNEY FOR JOICO

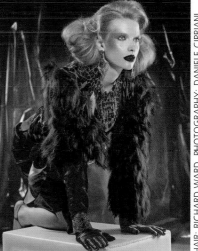

HAIR: RICHARD WARD, PHOTOGRAPHY: DANIELE CIPRIANI

EKU statement

GH4 (eku7) the range of protective equipment that should be available for clients

GH4 (eku8) the type of personal protective equipment available

EKU statement

GH4 (eku9) why it is important to use personal protective equipment

GH4 (eku10) how the position of your client and yourself can affect the desired outcome and reduce fatigue and the risk of injury

GH4 (eku11) why it is important to position your tools, products and materials for ease of use

GH4 (eku14) methods of working safely and hygienically and which minimise the risk of cross-infection and cross-infestation

GH4 (eku13) why it is important to keep your work area clean and tidy

GH4 (eku5) your own responsibilities under the current Control of Substances Hazardous to Health Regulations in relation to the use of colouring products

GH4 (eku6) what is contact dermatitis and how to avoid developing it whilst assisting with hair colouring services

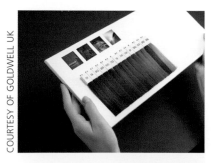

COURTESY OF GOLDWELL UK

A shade chart will help the client select the right colour

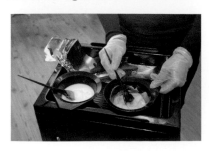

Mixing colours on a trolley

Maintaining personal hygiene standards

Review the section on washing positions in Chapter 5, Shampoo and condition hair, pages 74–5, for essential information on your standing position. For more information on preventing infection, avoiding dermatitis and personal health and hygiene, see Chapter 1, Make sure your own actions reduce risks to health and safety, pages 9–16.

Keeping the work area clean and safe to use at all times

Salon routines involving the work area are common throughout the Level 1 procedures. Please review this information by turning to Chapter 4, Prepare for hair services and maintain the work areas, pages 52–63, for more information.

Remember to keep the work area clean and tidy at all times. All waste items should be removed from the sinks and side area. This includes colouring foils, Easi-meche™ colour wraps, etc.; neck wool, plastic caps and cape; loose hair caught in the hair traps in the drain.

Activity

The table below shows the variety of colouring services that are available for clients, but not every salon or shop does them all. For the colouring services that take place in your shop, complete the missing information.

Service	Abbreviation used in the appointment system	What has to be prepared before the service?
re-growth or retouch colour		
full-head colour		
"T"-section highlights		
full head highlights		
cap highlights		
spot colour		

Disposal of waste

Colouring products create a lot of waste in and around the basin area. Unused, leftover colour or lightener should be washed out of colouring bowls as soon as the stylist has finished the service. These products swell up if left for any period of time and therefore need to be thoroughly rinsed away, as they form a sludge that might block the drains. Used foils and meches should be disposed of properly. Your salon may have its own procedures for this.

Activity

Write your answers to the following questions in your portfolio.

1 What is your salon's policy for protecting clients during colouring services?

2 What PPE is available for clients?

3 What PPE is available for you and when should you wear it?

4 What arrangements does your salon have for the disposal of waste items?

5 How would you know if a client was comfortable or not?

Remember

Any contact with chemical products is hazardous to health. Avoid developing dermatitis by always wearing disposable gloves.

For more information on **dermatitis**, see Chapter 1, Make sure your own actions reduce risks to health and safety.

Identifying when colours need reordering

Unlike regular shampoos and conditioners, the shampoos and conditioners used for colouring services are often not used as often. Keep checking on the levels of shampoos and conditioning products. Get used to gauging the weight of a full one as opposed to one that is nearly empty. Don't wait until they have run out; tell the stylist that stocks are running low and, if possible, go and get the refills out of stock and fill them as required.

EKU *statement*

GH4 (eku15) the importance of personal hygiene

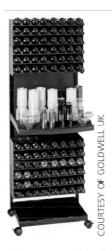

COURTESY OF GOLDWELL UK

Activity

Check your salon's procedure for maintaining stock levels of products and the ways in which the records are completed. Write this information in your portfolio for future reference.

For more information on replenishing basin products, see Chapter 5, Shampoo and condition hair.

When preparing the colour cart for the stylist, remember to take note if stocks are low

GH4.2   Remove colouring and lightening products

Minimising the risk of hair damage

Different colouring products work in different ways, so removing colours is not as straightforward as you might think. Different colour processes need to be handled differently, and this is especially true when two or more colours are to be removed. Lack of care and attention will ruin the result. You must know what to do and understand what is being done before attempting any colour removal. When hair has been coloured and lightened, it is in a far more delicate state than normal. You need to be particularly careful when you remove:

- highlight caps – apply surface conditioner to the highlights after rinsing and then gently comb through to reduce or eliminate stretching and reduce damage to the client's hair

EKU *statement*

GH4 (eku16) the importance of thoroughly rinsing products

EKU *statement*

GH4 (eku20) the types and causes of problems that may occur when removing colouring products and materials from the hair

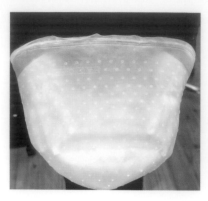

Highlight caps can stretch and damage the client's hair if not removed properly

EKU *statement*

GH4 (eku3) your own limits of authority for resolving colouring problems

GH4 (eku4) the person to whom you should report problems

GH4 (eku19) why it is important to follow manufacturers' and stylists' instructions and what might happen if they are not followed

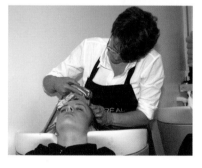

Always wear the recommended PPE when removing colours and foils!

EKU *statement*

GH4 (eku17) the importance of emulsifying permanent colouring products as part of the removal process

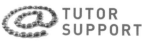

TUTOR SUPPORT

Task 7.2 Range of colours offered in the salon chart

- foils – highlighting foils are folded and cannot be pulled out of the hair without unfolding; you must carefully unfold them separately and rinse the colouring product on each one
- meches – many meches have a sticky edge that bonds on to the hair; these must not be pulled away from the lengths of the hair – they must be individually unwrapped and rinsed before they can be peeled away from the hair.

Colouring fault	Action to take
Colour on the client's skin	Remove with hair colour stain remover at the earliest possible moment.
Colour bleeding out of foils or meche on to other areas	Tell the stylist immediately so they can take corrective measures.
Colour not taken off properly	It may continue to develop or will affect any other following services – you must re-shampoo and condition.
Lightener or colour splashed onto the client or in their eyes	Give the client a dampened cotton wool wad and get help from a senior member of staff immediately.
Lightener or colour splashed onto the colouring gown	If possible, carefully replace the client's gown with a clean, fresh one; otherwise, sponge the stained area.

Remember

 Never remove all the foils at the same time. Ask the stylist for the correct order in which the colours must be removed.

EKU *statement*

GH4 (eku12) the safety considerations which must be taken into account when removing colouring products and materials

Keeping the client adequately protected

When you remove the hair colour, make sure that the client is adequately protected and take particular care not to get any water or colouring products on the client's skin or clothes. Any staining is unprofessional, and damage to clothes will probably have to be compensated for by the salon.

Emulsifying the colour

A shampoo will not spread evenly over the colour until it has been mixed with water; it releases the colour from the hair far easier after it has been emulsified. After adjusting the temperature, a small amount of water is sprinkled over the colour then, using the fingertips in a **rotary** massage technique, the colour blends together to form an emulsion. The massage is continued as this starts to release the residual colour from the hair, which can then be rinsed away.

Removal for a single colour process

The removal of single colours from the hair is similar to that of ordinary shampooing. However, special care should paid to removing colour around the hairline:

1 Sit the client at the basin and remove any caps, shoulder capes, etc.

2 Place a freshly laundered towel around the neck and across the shoulders.

3 Adjust the basin so that when the client's head is tilted back the position is comfortable with the minimum of towel supporting the neck. Put on your disposable gloves and apron.

4 Turn on the water and control the mixture of hot and cold. Test the temperature on the back of the hand to make sure it is neither too cold nor too hot.

5 Place one hand across the brow of the hairline, "damming" the water from splashing forward onto the face. Start rinsing the hair from the forehead, down either side, cupping the ears and through to the lengths.

6 Check the flow of water pressure and temperature regularly throughout.

7 Colours will come off the hair easier if they are **emulsified** first. So, during the rinsing process and before any shampooing takes place, gently massage the scalp and hair so that the water mixes with the colour to form an emulsion. Rinse this away.

8 Apply a small amount of the correct shampoo to the palms of the hand, lightly rub together and then apply evenly to the client's hair.

9 With the fingers clawed, massage the scalp (using the appropriate massage technique); cover the whole scalp making sure that no areas are missed.

10 Rinse the hair thoroughly, checking water temperature and pressure.

11 If the stylist requires two washes, repeat steps 8–10.

12 Rinse all traces of shampoo lather away from the hair and lightly squeeze out the excess water.

13 Condition the hair with an **anti-oxidant conditioner**.

Removing multiple colours

Removing highlights and slice colouring from the hair is more complex. If two or more colours are introduced to the hair, they are packaged separately in some way. There reasons for this are:

● different colours need to be kept apart so that they don't merge together, forming an unwanted effect

● different colours often develop at different rates, and therefore some might have been removed earlier than others

● the colouring technique involves specific positioning or placement; this maximises colour impact by using the shape texture and style of the hair

● sometimes the client's hair colour needs correcting, perhaps because of a previous poor application or because it has discoloured.

You need to know how to recognise different colours within the hair and how to remove them carefully and safely. Generally, for highlights or slice colouring with lighter and darker shades, remove the darkest shade first, then the next darkest and so on, because darker colours may run into lighter hair and ruin the effect. Bleach is often used to lighten

Remember

Never attempt to put colour-removing shampoo onto the hair before rinsing with water and emulsifying the product on the hair.

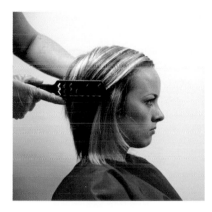

Use a vent brush to comb through new highlights to avoid stretching and damaging the hair

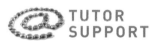

TUTOR SUPPORT

Task 7.3 Techniques used by the stylist when colouring the hair chart

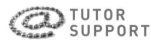

TUTOR SUPPORT

Discussion 7.1: Assist the stylist during the colour application and processing

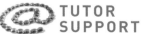

TUTOR SUPPORT

Task 7.4 Protecting ourselves and the client

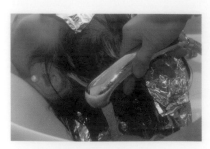

Remove colours in the order specified by the stylist

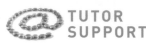

TUTOR SUPPORT

Task 7.7 Problems that could occur during the colour process

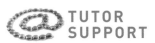

TUTOR SUPPORT

Discussion 7.2: Removing colour

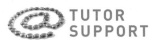

TUTOR SUPPORT

Task 7.6 List: Safety precautions when removing colour

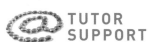

TUTOR SUPPORT

Task 7.5 Different types of colour are removed from the hair in different ways

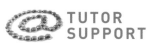

TUTOR SUPPORT

Short answer tests

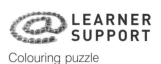

LEARNER SUPPORT

Colouring puzzle

hair and, during highlighting, certain areas can develop more readily than others; some sections will need to be removed earlier than others. The most important thing to remember is: if you don't know, ask. There will be a reason for colours to be removed in a specific order.

Activity

Answer the following questions.

1 Why should you emulsify the colour before shampooing off?
- it saves shampoo ☐
- it saves conditioner ☐
- it makes it easier to remove ☐
- it makes it stay on the hair better ☐

2 When taking off highlights, which colours are normaly removed first?
- the mid-tone colour ☐
- the darkest colour ☐
- the lightest colour ☐
- all at the same time ☐

3 When taking off highlights, which colours are normaly removed last?
- the mid-tone colour ☐
- the darkest colour ☐
- the lightest colour ☐
- all at the same time ☐

4 What effect do you think bleach will have in a set of high-lights?
- it makes the hair lighter ☐
- it makes the hair darker ☐
- it makes the hair blue ☐
- it makes the hair white ☐

5 Which product is easier to rinse out of the hair?
- semi-permanent colour ☐
- permanent colour ☐
- bleach ☐
- high-lift tint ☐

6 Who decides when a colour is ready for removal?
- you ☐
- the stylist ☐
- the manufacturer ☐
- the client ☐

Applying suitable conditioners

Depending on the type of colour used, you should now apply a suitable conditioner to improve the handling of the client's hair and smooth down the cuticle layer. For more information about the indicators of hair in good condition, see Chapter 6, Blow dry hair, page 87; for more information about conditioners and their beneficial effects on the hair, see Chapter 5, Shampoo and condition hair, pages 76–7.

The action of permanent colour on hair is stopped by the use of **anti-oxidant conditioners**. These are special conditioners that remove excess oxygen, which is released by the hydrogen peroxide during the colour service. If this residual oxygen is not removed, the free edges of the cuticle may not close down properly and may allow the newly introduced colour pigments to fade prematurely during future shampooing.

Leaving the client ready for further services

After completing the shampoo and conditioning processes, you should bring the client into an upright position and show them to a free styling unit. When they are seated, remove the towel and gently detangle the hair with a wide-tooth comb. Finally, squeeze any excess moisture from the hair and tell the stylist that their client is ready.

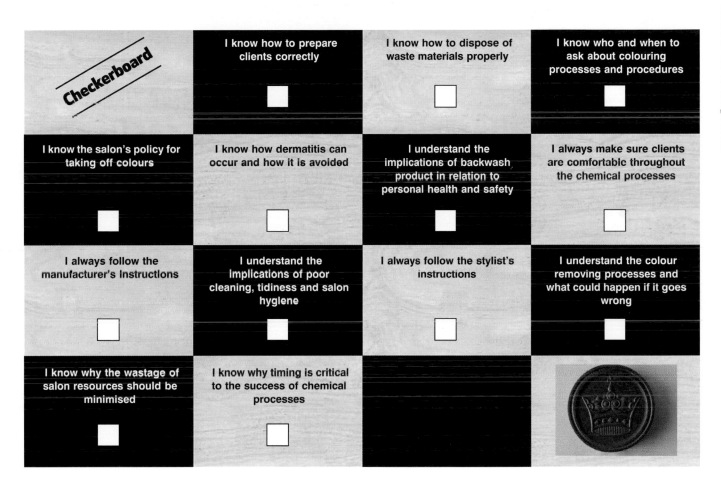

Revision questions

Q1 Fill in the blank: A semi-permanent colour will _____ during shampooing.

Q2 Natural hair that hasn't been coloured is called virgin hair. True or false?

Q3 Which of the following are natural pigments found within the hair? (You may choose more than one answer.)

1 paraphenylenediamine
2 pheomelanin
3 eumelanin
4 alpha keratin
5 beta keratin
6 henna

Q4 A lightener will remove natural pigments in hair. True or false?

Q5 Which of the following colours does not produce a regrowth? (Choose one answer.)

a semi-permanent
b quasi-permanent
c permanent
d lightener

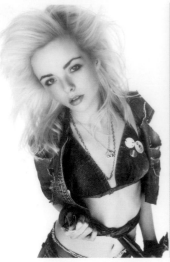

Chapter**eight**
Assist with perming hair services

GH5

GH5.1

GH5.2

**CREDIT VALUE
FOR UNIT GH5**
3 Credits

Unit title

GH5 Assist with perming hair services

This is an **optional** unit for Level 1. It is made up of 2 main outcomes.

Main outcomes

GH5 (eku1) Maintain effective and safe methods of working when assisting with perming services

GH5 (eku2) Neutralise hair as part of the perming process

Unit GH5: quick overview

What do I need to do for GH5.1?

You need to **prepare for neutralising** by:

- correctly protect and position the client and yourself
- keeping work areas clean and safe to use at all times
- maintaining personal hygiene standards
- reporting low neutralising products' stock

What do I need to do for GH5.2?

You need to **neutralise hair** by:

- neutralising (rebalancing the hair)
- preparing the neutraliser properly
- rinsing perm lotion from hair properly
- applying the neutraliser correctly
- applying a suitable conditioner

What things do I need to know?

You need to **know and understand**:

- your salon's way of preparing and protecting the clients
- your salon's procedures for the disposal of waste items
- your responsibilities in respect to COSHH
- to whom you should report problems
- what contact dermatitis is and how to avoid developing it

- how to clean and prepare the salon's work areas
- how to work safely and hygienically at all times
- the importance of neutralisers and the timing of processes
- the importance of rinsing the hair thoroughly
- the importance of following manufacturer's instructions
- the consequences of using the wrong neutraliser
- the problems that may occur during neutralising

Introduction

Perming is a process of permanently adding wave or curl to hair. Curlers are paced into a client's hair and perming solution is applied, changing the hair's natural structure. Curl development is checked and, when it is ready, the perming chemicals are rinsed from the hair. After towel drying **neutraliser** is applied, which fixes the movement into position.

The overall success of the perming service is in your hands!

Neutralising is a key process that is critical to the final effect.

Remember

Your salon will have its own way of neutralising that will be suited to the products it uses. Find out what it is and how you are expected to do it.

Keywords

Ammonium thioglycolate
an alkaline substance in perm lotions that reacts with the disulphide bonds

Disulphide bonds
the chemical bonds within the hair that are rearranged during perming and neutralising

Neutraliser
a chemical compound which is used to both balance and fix hair that has been previously permed

pH level
a measurement of a solution that denotes whether it is alkaline (pH 8–14), or acid (pH 6–1)

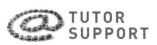

TUTOR SUPPORT

Task 8.6 List: Safety precautions when neutralising the hair

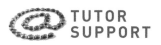

TUTOR SUPPORT

Task 8.2 Perm rods

GH5.1 Maintain effective and safe methods of working when assisting with perming services

Perming is a complex process. A satisfactory result can only be achieved if it is done correctly. The first part is wholly under the control of the stylist and, like a "relay race", the baton is now passed to you to finish what has been started without faltering and all in good time. First, it may help if you understand what is happening during the perming process.

EKU *statement*

GH5 (eku16) the role and importance of neutralisers in the perming process

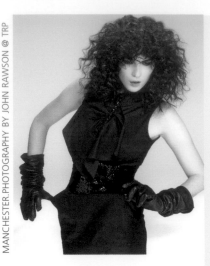

HAIR BY SHARON PEAKE @ ETHAS, MANCHESTER.PHOTOGRAPHY BY JOHN RAWSON @ TRP

Very curly permed hair can be luxurious and alluring

EKU *statement*

GH5 (eku1) your salon's requirements for client preparation

GH5 (eku7) the range of protective equipment that should be available for clients

GH5 (eku8) the type of personal protective equipment available

GH5 (eku9) why it is important to use personal protective equipment

GH5 (eku12) the safety considerations which must be taken into account when neutralising

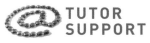

TUTOR SUPPORT

Task 8.1 Chart: Range of perms

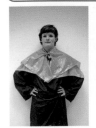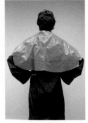

Ensure the gown you use is chemical proof, and top it off with a plastic cape

Science

Do you know how perms work?

The chemical reactions that take place within the hair during perming involve some complex chemistry that are covered in NVQ Levels 2 and 3. However, a simpler way of explaining the changes that take place within the hair during perming and neutralising is to use an illustration.

Imagine a wooden ladder

If you imagine that a ladder represents a single hair, the strength of the ladder is in the two long uprights. But when you climb the ladder, it flexes. So although it is strong and rigid, it is also capable of movement. The strength and shape of the ladder is derived from the rungs. Each rung is evenly spaced, holding the main structure of long uprights apart. These rungs are like the **disulphide bonds** in the hair shaft; they give natural hair its strength.

During perming, a solution of **ammonium thioglycolate** is added to the hair after the curlers have been wound in. The solution breaks the disulphide bonds chemically, just as if you had taken a saw and cut through all the rungs. So if you imagine that the ladder is now bent, the rungs now don't line up in the same places; the cut rungs have changed positions.

The next part of the perming process – neutralising – re-fixes the bonds by adding a solution enriched with oxygen. Just like the bent ladder, the rungs are now glued together in a new, reformed shape and – just like perming – if the gluing is done well, the ladder remains in a permanently bent shape. If it is done poorly, the ladder springs back to a straighter shape.

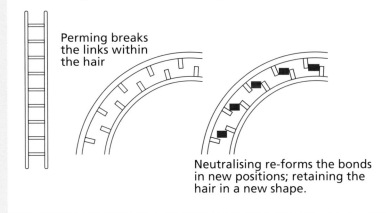

Perming breaks the links within the hair

Neutralising re-forms the bonds in new positions; retaining the hair in a new shape.

Correctly protect and position the client and yourself

Gowning the client

Because perm solutions are generally applied to hair by "post damping" (a method of pre-winding a perm and then applying the perm lotion after), the solutions tend to be very watery. This could be a hazard to the client unless adequate precautions are taken.

The majority of perm lotions are alkaline. Drips on fabric will be held against the skin like a poultice. This could cause irritation, swelling and even cause burns, and if it touches the client's clothes it may discolour the fabric. Make sure that the client is well protected. Put on a chemical-proof gown and secure a clean, fresh towel into place around their shoulders. Fix a plastic cape on top, ensuring that it is comfortable around the neck.

Protecting yourself

Your salon will provide all the personal protective equipment (PPE) that you may need in routine daily practices. Perming involves the handling and application of chemicals, so you must protect yourself from their potentially hazardous effects. Always read the manufacturers' instructions and follow the methods of practice that they specify. You are expected to wear and use the PPE provided for you. In the case of perming, these include disposable non-latex gloves and a water/splash-proof apron.

> **Activity**
>
> The Control of Substances Hazardous to Health (COSHH) Regulations 2003 explain the potential risks that hairdressing chemicals can have. Be aware of the information provided by the manufacturers about their handling, storage and safe disposal in your salon. As a general rule, perming products should be stored in an upright position and in a cool, dry place away from strong sunlight. Find out what the arrangements are in your salon and write these down in your portfolio for future reference.

> **Activity**
>
> **True or false**
>
> Neutraliser is used in a perm service to fix wave into hair.
>
> True ☐ False ☐
>
> You should always follow manufacturers' instructions when mixing chemicals.
>
> True ☐ False ☐
>
> Neutraliser is applied before rinsing.
>
> True ☐ False ☐
>
> Wearing disposable gloves helps to avoid developing dermatitis.
>
> True ☐ False ☐

Keeping work areas clean and safe to use at all times

Remove and dispose of waste items as soon as possible; don't leave cotton neck wool, plastic caps, etc. around the basins. Put them into a covered bin. Wash, dry and replace perm curlers back into the trays as soon as possible. Perming chemicals should be applied in a well-ventilated area. If there is any waste (some perming solutions cannot be saved for use another time), flush it down the basin with plenty of cold water.

Minimise waste

Get into the habit of eliminating waste. All the resources that you use cost money, and the only way that you can be more effective is to maximise your time and efforts whilst minimising the cost of carrying out your work.

Remember

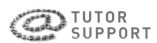

Barrier cream

Barrier cream is PPE for the client. It can be applied around the client's hairline and will help to prevent harm from chemicals during processing.

TUTOR SUPPORT

Task 8.4 Preparation for perming services

EKU statement

GH5 (eku2) your salon's and legal requirements for disposal of waste materials

GH5 (eku5) your own responsibilities under the current Control of Substances Hazardous to Health Regulations in relation to the use of neutralising products

GH5 (eku11) why it is important to position your tools, products and materials for ease of use

GH5 (eku13) why it is important to keep your work area clean and tidy

GH5 (eku19) the manufacturers' instructions for the specific neutralising products in your salon

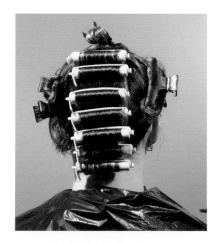

Once the perm curlers are in, ensure you apply the perming chemicals in a well-ventilated area

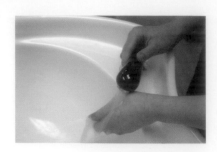

All businesses have metered water – running water down the drain costs money!

Remember

Perming products are chemically matched to the quantity and strengths of the neutralising solutions. If there is insufficient product, the perm will fail. If the top of the neutraliser has been left off, the solution will be too weak to work properly.

This can be illustrated further by thinking about what goes down the sink. Water is the first thing that comes to mind; cold water is a costly, but essential part of hairdressing. All business premises have metered water, so in principle every shampoo and conditioning rinse can be a calculated cost. Rinsing longer than necessary or leaving taps running between shampoos incurs unnecessary costs, especially if the water is hot. Cold incoming water is metered, and when you run hot water, you add the additional cost of heating it.

Remember

Dermatitis

Dermatitis is an occupational hazard for hairdressers; you reduce the risk by wearing vinyl gloves when using chemicals. They provide you with a guaranteed barrier against the action of harsh chemicals upon the skin. For more information on preventing infection, avoiding dermatitis and personal health and hygiene, see Chapter 1, Make sure your own actions reduce risks to health and safety, pages 12 and 20–1.

Maintaining personal hygiene standards

Your posture

Neutralising takes a lot longer than shampooing, so your standing position is particularly important. Review the sections on back and side wash positions in Chapter 5, Shampoo and condition hair, pages 68–9, so that you know and can avoid the risk of injury or a longer term back condition.

Reporting low neutralising products' stock

You are responsible for the neutralising process, and you will be the first to notice when neutralisers are running low, or containers have been left with their tops left off. The success of the perm is directly related to the chemical reaction of the neutraliser, so if too little or a defective product is used, then the perm won't work. Look at the condition and quantities of the products in stock and if the salon/shop is running low, tell someone who is responsible for stock reordering.

Be efficient and effective with your time

Always make good use of your time. There are always things to do in and around the salon/shop.

- clean work areas so that they are ready to receive clients
- prepare materials, look out for stock shortages and report them
- prepare the equipment, cleaning and washing the brushes, combs and curlers
- prepare client records, and get things ready for when they arrive
- prepare the trolleys, get the right curlers ready, make sure that the rubbers haven't perished and the end papers are at hand.

Activity

When you have a spare moment in the salon, separate the perm curlers into their different colour sizes. Check the condition of the perm rubbers and replace those that have perished or have gone over-elastic. When you have washed and dried them, separate them into bundles of 9 with a 10th curler around them, binding them together. You have now sorted the trolley trays into easily managed sizes and numbers!

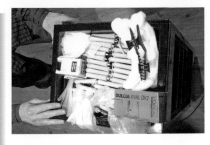

When you have some extra time, check that the trolleys are prepared

Choosing a neutraliser

Manufacturers produce matching perms and neutralisers. They are designed to work together and chemically balance each other out during the processes. Always use the matched lotions; many perms are now individually packed and you will find a perm lotion and its matched neutraliser in the box.

Some neutralisers may be supplied in bulk litre sizes as either a ready-to-use foaming liquid, or as one that needs to be accurately diluted with water. If you do use dilutions, always follow the manufacturer's instructions to get the right measurements and create the correct balance.

Activity

Answer the following questions in your portfolio:

1   Why is neutraliser an essential part to the perming process?

2   Why is timing a critical factor in the neutralising process?

Remember

Some neutralisers can be applied directly from the container, whereas others are applied with a sponge from a colouring bowl.

EKU *statement*

GH5 (eku3) your own limits of authority for resolving neutralising problems

GH5 (eku17) the importance of accurate timing when neutralising perms

GH5 (eku18) the importance of thoroughly rinsing neutralisers

GH5 (eku19) the manufacturers' instructions for the specific neutralising products in your salon

GH5 (eku20) why it is important to follow manufacturers' and stylists' instructions and what might happen if they are not followed

GH5.2   Neutralise hair as part of the perming process

Neutralising (rebalancing the hair)

Neutralising is the process of fixing the curl or movement into the hair and returning it to a balanced chemical state. An industry term, "neutralising" is a little misleading. In chemistry, a "neutral" chemical condition is neither acidic nor alkaline (pH 7.0). However, in hairdressing, the "neutralising" treatment returns the previously processed hair to the hair and skin's healthy, but slightly acidic, natural state of pH 5.5.

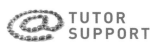

TUTOR SUPPORT

Task 8.3 Tools and equipment found on the perm trolley

Remember

 Rebalancing the pH of the hair is essential for maintaining hair in good condition. If the hair is not rebalanced, the hair will be dry, porous and the perm will be very difficult to manage afterwards.

Remember

 Check that the client is comfortable and that towels support the client's neck form a barrier, preventing water from running down the back of their neck. Back wash basins are preferable because it is easier to keep the drips of chemicals away from the client's eyes.

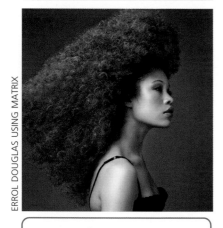

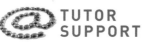
TUTOR SUPPORT

Task 8.5 Critical time factors in perming

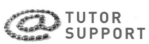
TUTOR SUPPORT

Discussion 8.1: Assist the stylist during the perm winding, solution application and processing

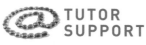
TUTOR SUPPORT

Task 8.7 Perming problems

Preparing the neutraliser properly

What must you prepare before you neutralise a perm? Neutralising always takes place at the basin, so any plastic caps, capes or cotton wool must be carefully removed and any damp towels must be replaced.

Preparation beforehand

1 Gather together the materials you will need.
2 Make sure there is a back wash basin free.

Rinsing perm lotion from hair properly

Rinsing with warm water removes the perming chemicals from the hair and stops any further processing. When you rinse you must take special care not to dislodge any of the curlers or rods.

First rinsing

1 As soon as the perm is complete, move the client immediately to the back wash basin. Make sure they are comfortable.
2 Carefully remove the cap. The hair is in a soft and weak stage at this point, so don't put unnecessary tension on it. Leave the curlers in place.
3 Run the water. You need an even supply of warm water. The water must be neither hot nor cold, as this will be uncomfortable for the client. Hot water will also irritate the scalp and could burn. Check the pressure and temperature against the back of your hand. Remember that your client's head may be sensitive after the perming process.
4 Rinse the hair thoroughly with the warm water. This may take about 5 minutes, or longer if the hair is long. It is this rinsing that stops the perm process – until you rinse away the lotion, the hair will still be processing. Direct the water away from the client's eyes and the face.
5 Make sure you rinse **all** the client's hair, including the nape curlers. If a curler slips out, gently wind the hair back onto it immediately.

Applying the neutraliser correctly

After rinsing, blot the saturated hair with a dry towel until it is just slightly damp. Prepare and apply the correct neutraliser (following the manufacturer's instructions) and leave on for the appropriate length of time.

Applying neutraliser

1 Make sure your client is in a comfortable sitting position.
2 Blot the hair thoroughly, using a towel (you may need more than one).

3 When no surplus water remains, apply the neutraliser. Follow the manufacturer's instructions. These may tell you to pour the neutraliser through the hair, or apply it with a brush or sponge, or use the spiked applicator bottle. Some foam neutralisers need to be pushed briskly into the hair. Make sure that neutraliser comes into contact with all of the hair on the curlers.

4 When all the hair has been covered, time the process according to the instructions. The usual time is 5 to 10 minutes.

5 Gently and carefully remove the curlers. Don't pull or stretch the hair. It may still be soft, especially towards the ends, and you don't want to disturb the curl formation.

6 Apply the neutraliser to the hair again, covering all the hair. Arrange the hair so that the neutraliser does not run over the face. Leave for the time recommended, usually another 5 to 10 minutes.

Second rinsing

1 Run the water, again checking temperature and pressure.

2 Rinse the hair thoroughly to remove the neutraliser.

3 You can now treat the hair with an after-perm (anti-oxidant) or conditioner. Use the one recommended by the manufacturer of the perm and neutraliser, to be sure that the chemicals are compatible.

Applying a suitable conditioner

Perm aids or conditioner and balanced conditioners (anti-oxidants) help neutralise the effect of the chemical process by helping to restore the pH balance of the hair to pH 5.5 and smooth down the hair cuticle, improving the hair's look, feel, combability and handling. At the end of the neutralising process, you will have returned the hair to a normal, stable state.

After the perm

Bring the client into an upright position and show them to a free styling unit. When they are seated, remove the towel and gently detangle the hair with a wide toothed comb. Finally, squeeze any excess moisture from the hair and tell the stylist that their client is ready.

Perming and neutralising faults

The following table highlights the sorts of problems that can occur during perming and neutralising. Many of the faults are created in the perming part of the process and have been left in to show how many things can go wrong. However, the possible causes that are created by poor/incorrect neutralising and not following the manufacturer's instructions are indicated with a star (*). Always tell the stylist if you see or think you have an unexpected result.

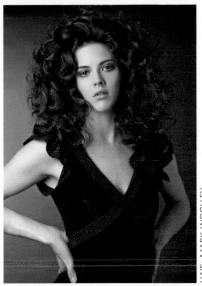

HAIR: MARK WOOLLEY

Remember

When applying a conditioner, apply to the palms of the hands first and gently work the conditioner through the hair. Do not massage the scalp or pull or comb the hair because it may soften the newly formed curl.

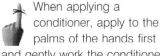

PROTIP

Use a wide toothed comb such as this one to detangle hair after perming

EKU statement

GH5 (eku4) the person to whom you should report problems

GH5 (eku20) why it is important to follow manufacturers' and stylists' instructions and what might happen if they are not followed

GH5 (eku21) what might happen if the correct neutralising agent is not applied

GH5 (eku22) the types and causes of problems that may occur when neutralising perms

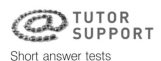

TUTOR SUPPORT

Short answer tests

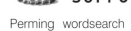

LEARNER SUPPORT

Perming wordsearch

Fault	Possible cause
scalp is tender, sore or broken	curlers were too tight
	wound curlers rested on the skin
	lotion was spilt on the scalp
	* there was cotton wool padding soaked with chemicals between the curlers
	hair was pulled tightly
	perm was over-processed
hair is broken	hair was wound too tightly
	curlers were secured too tightly
	* incorrect chemicals were used
	hair was over-processed
	chemicals in the hair reacted with the lotion
hair is straight	* wrong neutralising lotion was used for the type of hair
	hair was under-processed
	curlers were too large for the hair length
	* neutralising wasn't done properly
	* rinsing was inadequate
	conditioners used before perming were still on the hair
	hair was coated and resistant to the lotion
hair is frizzy	lotion was too strong for hair of this texture
	winding was too tight
	curlers were too small
	hair was over-processed
	* neutraliser wasn't diluted
	* neutralising wasn't done properly
	there are fish-hooks
perm is weak and drops	* lotion was applied unevenly
	* neutraliser was too dilute
	* neutralising was poorly done
	* hair was stretched while soft
	curlers or sections were too large
some hair sections are straight	curler angle was wrong
	curlers were placed incorrectly
	curlers were too large
	sectioning or winding was done carelessly
	* neutraliser was not applied correctly

Activity

What is the most likely perm outcome to occur from poor neutralising? How could you make sure that this doesn't happen to you? Write your answers in your portfolio.

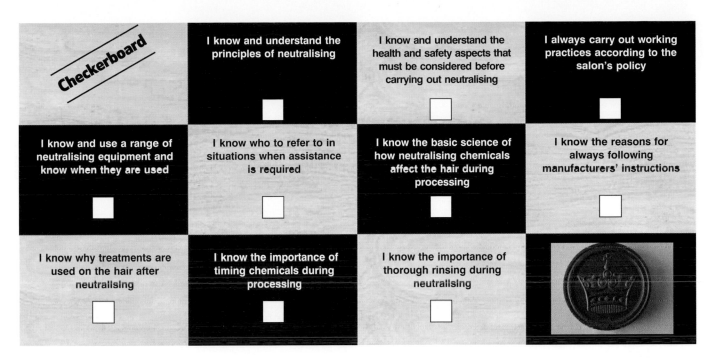

Checkerboard	I know and understand the principles of neutralising ☐	I know and understand the health and safety aspects that must be considered before carrying out neutralising ☐	I always carry out working practices according to the salon's policy ☐
I know and use a range of neutralising equipment and know when they are used ☐	I know who to refer to in situations when assistance is required ☐	I know the basic science of how neutralising chemicals affect the hair during processing ☐	I know the reasons for always following manufacturers' instructions ☐
I know why treatments are used on the hair after neutralising ☐	I know the importance of timing chemicals during processing ☐	I know the importance of thorough rinsing during neutralising ☐	

Revision questions

Q1　Fill in the blank: Neutraliser is a chemical that is used to _____ the curl into previously permed hair.

Q2　The post-damping method requires the perm to be wound first. True or false?

Q3　Which of the following pH values would indicate an acidic tendency? (You may choose more than one answer.)

　　1　4　　　　　　　　　**4**　7
　　2　5　　　　　　　　　**5**　8
　　3　6　　　　　　　　　**6**　9

Q4　The COSHH regulations cover the legal requirements for handling chemical products. True or false?

Q5　Which of the following PPE is made available for your benefit? (Choose one answer.)

　　a　gown　　　　　　　**c**　vinyl gloves
　　b　towel　　　　　　　**d**　plastic cape

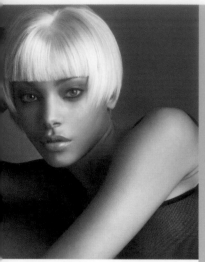

Chapter**nine**
Plait and twist hair using basic techniques

ERROL DOUGLAS USING MATRIX, PHOTOGRAPHY ANDREW O'TOOLE

GH6

GH6.1

GH6.2

CREDIT VALUE FOR UNIT GH6
4 Credits

Unit title

GH6 Plait and twist hair using basic techniques

This is an **optional** unit for Level 1. It is made up of 2 main outcomes.

Main outcomes

GH6 (eku1) Maintain effective and safe methods of working when plaiting and twisting

GH6 (eku2) Plait and twist hair

Unit GH6: quick overview

What do I need to do for GH6.1?

You need to **prepare for plaiting and twisting** by:

● correctly protect and position clients and yourself

● keeping work areas clean at all times

● maintaining personal hygiene standards

● completing the service efficiently

What do I need to do for GH6.2?

You need to **plait and twist hair** by:

● preparing the client

● controlling your tools

● securing the free ends of plaits

● learning about hair textures

● maintaining an even tension

● applying suitable products

● checking clients' comfort and satisfaction

● creating loose hanging plaits

● making French plaits and twists

● applying twisting techniques

What things do I need to cover?

You will using:

● sprays, serums and gels

You will be creating:

● cornrows, French plaits and 2-strand twists

What things do I need to know?

You need to **know and understand**:

- your salon's way of preparing and protecting the clients
- what contact dermatitis is and how to avoid developing it
- how to work safely and hygienically at all times
- why you should work in a tidy and ordered way
- why you should use professional bands to secure the hair
- why you should follow the stylist's instructions
- the consequences of excess tension on hair and the indicators of traction alopecia
- how to prepare and cleanse the hair
- how the hair texture affects your options for styling
- why even sectioning and tensioning is important
- the products that are suitable for the styles and how they should be used

Introduction

Plaiting and twisting hair requires a great deal of patience, repeated practice and perseverance. The skills that you will learn will not be wasted.

Plaiting and twisting is fun and the effects are exciting!

These techniques or manual dexterity underpin many other hairdressing procedures.

Keywords

Traction alopecia
a condition that is caused by the excessive pulling of hair at the root, it is often associated with longer hair worn in plaits, twists, hair-ups and extensions

Practice block
a modelling head with longer hair that can be attached to a work surface for practicing techniques

Cornrows
(also known as cane rows) a term used to describe an effect created by multiple rows of plaits that follow the contour of the head

French plait
(also known as Congo plait/ Guinea plait) a 3-strand plait that starts, centrally, near the front hairline and continues closely to the scalp to the nape and continues as a freely hanging plait beyond

Senegalese twists
a twisting technique that resembles the plaited effect created by cornrows

| GH6.1 | Maintain effective and safe methods of working when plaiting and twisting |

Plaiting and twisting is something that can be practised whenever you have any free time. You can try out different designs and ways of doing things on a **practice block** until you have perfected your techniques. The most important thing to remember with any longer hair work is to have a plan of what you are trying to

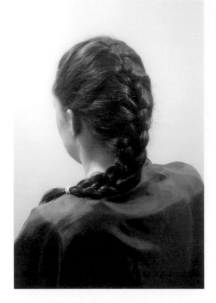

You can practise plaiting techniques whenever you have spare time

HTTP://TRENDYNEWHAIRSTYLES.BLOGSPOT.COM

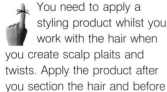

Cornrows are an intricate, attractive and highly detailed modern classic

Remember

You need to apply a styling product whilst you work with the hair when you create scalp plaits and twists. Apply the product after you section the hair and before you position the plait or twist.

achieve before you start. The NVQ Level 1 standards require the student to be able to perform 2 forms of plaiting technique and 1 type of twist. The 2 forms of plaiting techniques are:

1 a free-hanging plait comprising 3 stems or strands to produce the **French plait** (also known as Congo plait/Guinea plait)

2 a close "head hugging" design made up of several scalp plaits known as **cornrows** (also known as cane rows).

The French plait is a simple but attractive way of wearing longer hair down, secured but not loose. In hairdressing terms, it falls into what we call "hair-ups" – many clients tend to have French plaits for specific occasions such as weddings, parties and formal evenings out. Clients with long hair (and hair extensions) can display the length of their hair whilst having it controlled; it is often finished off with a themed decoration with some form of hair ornament.

Cornrows have become a popular way of wearing finely detailed scalp plaits that can form straight, curved or zig zag patterns; swirls, circles and wavy designs. The techniques were originally produced by African tribes to define their identities, but have become a popular option for any hair type. Good cornrowing is intricate, attractive, highly detailed and long lasting, and the technique is quickly becoming a modern classic.

The NVQ Level 1 standards also require you to be able to produce twisted hair effects that have 2 stems. These 2 stem twists are known as **double twists** and, like cornrows, originate from Africa. Gel and pomade are used together to bond the twist as it is formed, creating head hugging designs very similar to cornrows, or "off-the-head" effects for more "quirky" fashionable looks.

 Activity

Any long hair design work needs to be planned from the outset. Choose either a plaiting technique or a twisting technique. Research different effects that can be achieved by using this technique in different ways. Use style magazines and websites to find and gather the information. After collecting together images and sketches of what you would like to do, choose one effect that you would like to re-create.

Prepare a practice block by washing, drying, conditioning and detangling the hair. When it is ready, practise the techniques. When you have finished, take photos of the finished effects for your portfolio.

Correctly protect and position clients and yourself

The client's hair has to be shampooed and, if necessary, conditioned as well as dried before you can start the styling service. So, after you have put a clean, fresh gown on the client, place a clean towel around their shoulders before moving them to the basin. Check which products you should be using with the stylist and shampoo and prepare the hair as outlined in Chapter 5, Shampoo and condition hair, page 74. On returning to the styling unit, prepare the hair by:

- detangling (remember to work through the point ends first and then work back up the hair to nearer the root)

- blow drying with a flat brush to keep the hair as smooth as possible
- making sure that the client is comfortable and getting the stylist to check that the hair is ready for the service.

When you are ready to start, ask the stylist if you should place a plastic cape around the client instead of a towel. Many plaiting and twisting techniques use products like hair glazes, sprays, gels, waxes and pomades. You need to keep both the styling gown and client clean throughout the process, so it may be easier to cover the client's shoulders and clothes at the beginning.

A full head of scalp plaits or twists takes a long time to complete. The main health and safety concerns relate to the length of time that you will be standing whilst doing the work, and the client's comfort, positioning and protection during the process. You can review the information relating to posture whilst standing in Chapter 1, Make sure your own actions reduce risks to health and safety, page 21.

Keeping work areas clean at all times

Prepare all of the equipment and products that you need beforehand and put them on your trolley. Professional bands for plaits and twists, the products that you will be using, and combs, brushes, sectioning clips, etc. should be all cleaned, sterilised and made ready for use. For more information on cleaning, sterilisation and general salon hygiene, see Chapter 1, Make sure your own actions reduce risks to health and safety, pages 9–21.

Activity
Preparing for plaiting and twisting hair
Complete this activity by filling in the missing information in the table below.

Preparation	What do you need to do?
client	
yourself	
tools/materials	

Maintaining personal hygiene standards

Everything that comes into contact with the client's skin or hair must be clean and hygienic. Similarly, your own personal standards of health and hygiene should not present any risk to the client. This will prevent the risk of cross-infection and helps to maintain a healthy safe environment. For more information on preventing infection and personal health and hygiene, see Chapter 1, Make sure your own actions reduce risks to health and safety, pages 14–15 and 20.

Remember

Plaiting and twisting takes a long time, so both you and the client need to be comfortable throughout the service.

EKU *statement*

GH6 (eku3) what is contact dermatitis and how to avoid developing it whilst plaiting and twisting hair

GH6 (eku11) the importance of personal hygiene

GH6 (eku12) methods of cleaning, disinfecting and/or sterilisation used in salons

Remember

 Plaiting and twisting is intricate work. If your tension on the hair starts to relax, it will be noticeable at the end. You need to pay attention to this and fix it as you go along.

Remember

You need to operate like a professional, so if you are given the responsibility to do the service on a client, it must be up to standard.

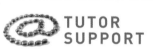 **TUTOR SUPPORT**

Task 9.1 List: Health and safety

Completing the service efficiently

Different salons have their own ways of doing things, each with its own appointment scheduling system. Working on the client may seem like a real treat for you, but remember that both the client and the stylist have other things to do as well:

- if you have problems with the client's hair, **stop** and get help – don't progress further as it may have a "knock-on" effect on the whole style and the client may need to be started all over again
- keep an eye on the time so that you don't overrun or make the client late.

The following table provides a rough guideline for how long each type of work will take:

Length	French plait	cornrows (10 rows)	twists (10 scalp twists)	twists (40 off the head)
shoulder length at one length	20 minutes	1½ hours	1 hour	2–2½ hours
beyond shoulder at one length	25 minutes	2 hours	1½ hours	
short layered length 10–15 cm		1½ hours	1½ hours	1½ hours
mid-length layered		1½ hours	1½ hours	2 hours
long layered	25 minutes	2 hours	1½ hours	2 hours

Remember

 Listen to the stylist: they know the best way to tackle the hair.

GH6.2 Plait and twist hair

EKU *statement*

GH6 (eku14) the importance of following your stylist's instructions

Preparing the client

Although you are styling the client's hair, you are doing it under the direct supervision of the stylist. They are ultimately responsible for what you do, and therefore you must follow their instructions and wishes throughout the plaiting or twisting service. Only use the styling products that they have asked you to use, and complete the work in the sequence of steps that they give you. For instance, if they have specifically said that they want you to start at the front hairline and to work back from there in to the rest of the hair, then that is where you must start.

Controlling your tools

You must work in a controlled way. Carefully divide the hair and secure the areas that you are not yet working on out of the way. Be careful with the clips that you use because they can catch on the hair and leave it looking untidy, frizzy, or even snap it. It is impossible to replace untidy lengths of hair once they have been separated from the main stems of hair. If this happens, the inexperienced stylist will make it worse by trying to overload the hair with a styling product to hide the mistake.

Remember

Plaiting and twisting is a step-by-step procedure; if you miss one out it will impact the rest of the style.

EKU *statement*

GH6 (eku19) how hair texture affects the plaiting process and styling possibilities

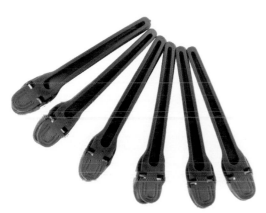

A flat clip: the correct clip to use to divide and secure hair for sectioning

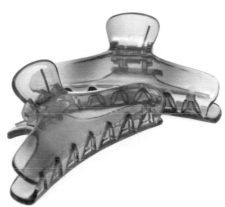

NEVER use a crocodile clip!

Remember

Flat-jawed clips are easier to work with than "spiky" crocodile clips. Flat clips will keep the sections of hair that you are not yet working on smooth. They will stop the hair from bulking out and eliminate the problems of crimped hair. Crimped hair is caused by haphazard sectioning and twisting of the hair in a way that it wouldn't normally lie.

Ideally, for styles that require a smooth, sleek effect on the hair, never clip hair in to a position above the horizontal. This causes the root area to lift, and affects the way that the hair will lie after you take it down and want to work with it.

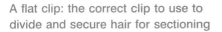

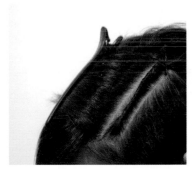

Good sectioning: smooth and flat, with the correct clips

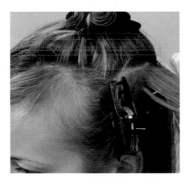

Bad sectioning: hair lifted above the horizontal, the wrong sort of clips used

EKU *statement*

GH6 (eku13) the importance of using bands for professional use

GH6 (eku22) methods of securing the completed plait and twists

GH6 (eku19) how hair texture affects the plaiting process and styling possibilities

Securing the free ends of plaits

As cornrows and scalp twists extend beyond the contour of the head, the freely hanging lengths can be secured:

- temporarily, whilst you work through the style, with Kirby grips
- to finish nearer to the head, by sewing with thread using a curved needle (See Chapter 10, Remove hair extensions, page 142) or by using professional bands to allow the remainder of the hair to be styled in some other way
- to finish the ends of the plait or twist, using professional bands to enable the freely hanging plaits/twists to created an overall braided effect.

Remember

Always use professional bands because these will be less damaging to the client's hair than using any other type of elastic or rubber band.

EKU statement

GH6 (eku23) how to handle the hair when plaiting and twisting to maintain a correct and even tension

GH6 (eku21) the importance of sectioning hair accurately when plaiting and twisting

Remember

 Always detangle the hair and brush it through as you work through each section or stem of hair.

EKU statement

GH6 (eku24) how to adjust the tension of plaits

EKU statement

GH6 (eku25) the types of products available for use with plaits and twists and when you would use them

GH6 (eku26) the importance of using products economically

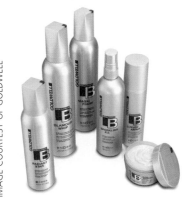

There is a huge range of styling and finishing products available

Learning about hair textures

The choice of final styling will be made by the stylist and will be based on the texture of the hair. Certain hair textures suit specific styling, for example, a head of cornrows on African Caribbean hair is probably better finished in free hanging plaits rather than with heat styling. Alternately, European hair may be slippery and will need to be well secured.

Straight hair is easier to style in plaits rather than twists, whereas curly hair can be cornrowed or twisted. Freely hanging ends of scalp plaits or twists can be crimped, waved, curled or worn as a blown-out "Afro".

Maintaining an even tension

The stylist will provide you with the necessary instructions because they know the best way of completing the work to achieve a satisfactory result. Any deviation will probably cause your styling to go wrong and possibly leave you with a very unhappy client.

Be careful with your tensioning as you handle and manipulate the hair. Obviously you don't want to hurt the client or damage their hair, but you do need to maintain an even pressure so that the hair lies properly in the design. If hair starts to "bulk out" within a plait whilst you are working on it, unravel it and do the plait again – it won't get any better the longer you leave it. It actually gets worse!

If a client says that the plait or twist is pulling and painful, you have to ease the stress on the root of the hair that is pulling at the scalp. First of all, find the area that is the problem. This may show as tension and lifting at the scalp. Then decide whether the end of a tail comb can ease and loosen the stem of hair, or whether you have to undo and start that plait again.

Don't waste your time and energy

When you encounter problems with the technique that you are trying to apply, **stop**. Get your stylist to help or give you some advice on how to tackle the problem. A lot of plaiting and twisting work is incremental; that means that everything is done in an ordered, progressive way. This means that you need to do **A** before **B** and **B** before **C,** etc. If something goes wrong at **B** and you don't sort it out then and carry on to finish, you may not be able to correct it without having to undo steps **Z** back to **C** – and that may be hours of work!

Applying suitable products

There is an ever-growing range of styling and finishing products available to the profession, which can be confusing. The products that you will need to use work in the following ways. They can:

- provide hold, whilst you work, by bonding the hair together
- finish the hair, improving the look and feel
- provide a final hold, bonding the finished hairstyle in place.

Quite simply, a hairstyle that is designed to last for a longer time, such as scalp plaits, scalp twists and off-the-head twists, needs a fixative to hold and to prolong the durability of the hairstyle; whereas a hairstyle like a French plait needs to look smooth, shiny and elegant. There are 2 main forms of hair product that you will be using:

- **styling products**, such as gels and pomades, which contain fixatives to hold and support the hair in its shape whilst you are handling the hair giving it definition and shape
- **finishing products**, such as serums and sprays, which can add shine and lustre to improve the look of the hair or provide a final fix.

The choice of what you use should be made by the stylist, as they will know what effect they are trying to achieve and what will work best with the hair. Products like wax, serum or gel come in what seems like relatively small containers. This is because these products are highly concentrated and a very small amount goes a long way. Always use these products sparingly because it is easy to overload the hair – if you do, it may need to be rewashed and the styling re started! It is also poor economy, as these products are expensive and it is a waste of the salon's resources.

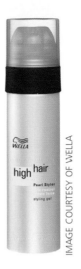

Gel is ideal for styling whilst you handle the hair

Styling products

Product	Suitability	Purpose	Application	If overapplied
dry wax	suitable for bonding the ends of **cornrows** and **twists**	moderately firm hold providing a non-wet look or greasy finish	applied in small amounts with the fingertips into ends of the hair	easy to add too much and overload the hair, particularly on finer hair types
normal (grease-based) wax	suitable for bonding the lengths and ends of **cornrows** and **twists**	firm hold; high definition and texture with a moist or slightly wet-look effect	applied in small amounts with the fingertips into lengths of the hair during the initial separation of strands	easy to add too much and overload the hair, particularly on finer hair types
hair gel	suitable for bonding the lengths and ends of **cornrows** and **twists**	wet look effect with very strong hold when gel dries into position	applied with fingertips or comb; it is easy to see where it has been missed	you can't overload the hair as the look is based on 100% coverage
styling glaze	suitable for bonding the lengths and ends of **cornrows**	wet-look effect with firm–strong hold when it dries into position	applied first to the hands and rubbed into the hair all over; plait the hair; apply more if it dries	you can't overload the hair as the look is based on 100% coverage
serum	suitable for **French plaits**	improves handling, provides shine; smoothes out frizzies whilst plaiting	applied in small amounts with the finger tips into pre-plaited hair	it is easy to overload the hair, making it greasy
fixing sprays – mild, moderate and firm hold	**plaits** and **twists**	used as a final fixative or as a styling product if scrunched into "fanned" ends	applied to pre-dried hair by directional spraying from 30 cm away	too much will make hair "crunchy"

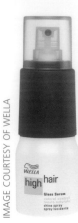

IMAGE COURTESY OF WELLA

Serum will add lustre and fix a finished style

EKU *statement*

GH6 (eku15) the potential consequences of excessive tension on the hair

GH6 (eku16) what is traction alopecia

GH6 (eku17) how to identify the signs of traction alopecia

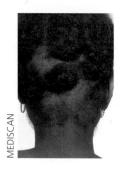

MEDISCAN

This is what traction alopecia looks like

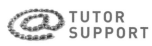

TUTOR SUPPORT

Task 9.2 The tools and equipment needed for plaiting and twisting

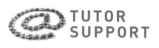

TUTOR SUPPORT

Task 9.3 Styling products chart

Remember

Always follow the manufacturer's instructions and guidance for use when using any styling or finishing products.

Checking clients' comfort and satisfaction

Plaiting or twisting services require that the client be seated in the same position for a long time – at least you can move around. Stop now and again to give yourself and the client a break. Check with the client to make sure that what you are doing is okay and not painful. They may not want to say anything, or speak out; it's your job to ask. Make a point of asking at least 3 or 4 times during a full head of scalp plaits or twists and 2 or 3 times for a partial head. If you put excessive pressure and tension on the client's hair then you could cause **traction alopecia**.

Traction alopecia

One of the more serious after-effects of wearing hair in any scalp plaited or scalp twisted hairstyle is traction alopecia. This occurs when constant pressure is exerted upon the roots of the hair. This can result in hair loss in patches on the scalp, showing as baldness, and is particularly obvious in areas of weaker hair such as the temples or hairlines.

If the client tells you that they have an unpleasant tightness in any area as you are working, try releasing the pressure by using the pointed end of a tail comb to ease the stems of the plaits. If this does not release the tension, you will have to remove the plait or twist and re-start that area again.

Remember

If there is an imbalance in the tension of the strands whilst you plait, see if you can even it out by carefully lifting the tightest with the end of a tail comb.

Creating loose hanging plaits

Plaiting is a method of intertwining three or more strands of hair to create a variety of woven hairstyles. When this work is done for specific occasions, it is often accompanied by ornamentation: fresh flowers, glass or plastic beads, coloured silks and added hair are popular. The numerous options for plaited effects are determined by the following factors:

● number of plaits or twists used

● positioning of the plait or twist across the scalp or around the head

● the way in which the plaits are made (under or over)

● any ornamentation/decoration or added hair applied.

Remember

"Plaits" usually refers to a free-hanging stem(s) of hair that is left to show hair length. This length can be natural or can be extended by adding hair during the plaiting process; an example is the "French" or "fish tail" plait.

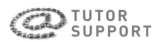

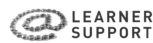

Short answer tests

LEARNER SUPPORT

Plaiting puzzle

Loose plaiting (3-stem loose plait)

The 3-stem plait is easily achieved and demonstrates the basic principle of plaiting hair.

1 Divide the hair to be plaited into 3 equal sections.
2 Hold the hair with both hands, using your fingers to separate the sections.
3 Starting from either the left or the right, place the outside section over the centre one. Repeat this from the other side.
4 Continue placing the outside sections of hair over the centre ones until you reach the ends of the stems.
5 Secure the free ends with thread or professional band.

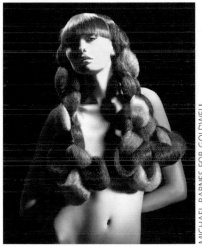

MICHAEL BARNES FOR GOLDWELL

Remember

The tension used in plaiting can exert exceptional pressure on the hair follicle. Scalp-type plaits/cornrows are more vulnerable than free-hanging plaits. In extreme cases, this may cause hair loss; areas of hair become thin and baldness may even result! **Traction alopecia** is particularly obvious at the temples of younger girls with long hair who regularly wear their hair tied up for school, sport or dancing.

Step-by-step: 3-stem "French" plaiting

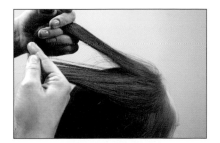

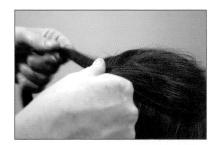

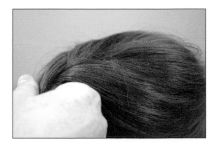

Step 1 Brush the hair to remove all tangles. With the hair tilted backwards, divide the foremost hair into 3 equal sections.

Step 2 Starting from either the left or the right, cross an outside stem over the centre stem. Repeat this action with the opposite outer stem.

Step 3 Section a fourth stem (smaller in thickness than the initial 3 stems) and incorporate this with the next outside stem you are going to cross.

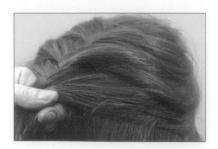

Step 4 Cross this thickened stem over the centre, and repeat this step with the opposite outer stem.

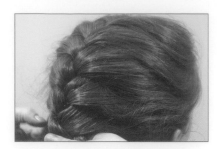

Step 5 Continue this sequence of adding hair to the outer stem before crossing it over the centre.

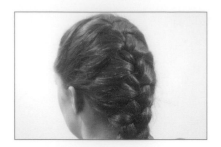

Step 6 When there is no more hair to be added, continue plaiting down to the ends and secure them with a professional band.

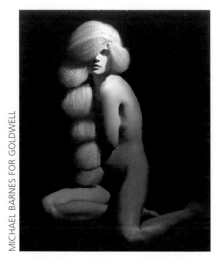

MICHAEL BARNES FOR GOLDWELL

Making French plaits and twists

The cornrow is, like the 2 examples above, a type of 3-stem plait. However, it is secured closer to the scalp, to create head-hugging patterned designs that can last for 3 or 4 weeks. Cornrows (also known as "cane rows") originated in Africa and have been a unique way of displaying hair art and design, often incorporating complex patterns indicating status or tribal connection. In fact, as this art form has been passed down for thousands of years, it is quite probable that the very first hairdressers worked on these elaborate techniques.

Cornrows create design patterns across the scalp by working along predefined channels of hair. These channels are secured to the scalp by interlocking each of the 3 subdivided stems as the plaiting technique progresses. Short or even layered hair can be made to look longer if extension hair is added during the process. The added hair is plaited into the style along each of the sections that create the plaited effect.

When cane rows have been applied to the hair, the effect can last up to 6 weeks or more before they should be removed. Advice should be given on handling and maintaining the hair, although regular shampooing can still be carefully achieved.

Shampoo and condition the hair

The hair must be shampooed, and possibly conditioned, before plaiting or twisting. You need to make sure that any traces of product – moisturisers, gels, sheens and oils – are removed from the hair first. These products often leave a sticky or oily residue that can be made worse when applied to previously plaited hair, if the product build-up has not been removed each time.

Drying into shape

Both plaiting and twisting techniques tend to make the hair appear shorter; with plaits, much of the original length is used laterally (across and around the head) as decoration. Blow dry the hair first, to make the most of its overall length. This is necessary anyway, as the hair needs to be dried and made smoother before any other work can take place. After blow drying, the hair and scalp can be prepared with hair oils or dressings. Any moisturising will be beneficial to the hair, making it more elastic, improving any brittleness and making it more flexible.

Remember

Hair products designed especially for these services are often very different to the everyday styling products you would use in other styling services. Use these products in line with manufacturer's instructions and be careful not to overload the hair during the styling process. When the product has been applied to the hair it will be difficult to remove it without re-washing!

Step-by-step cornrowing

Step 1 Wash, condition and pre-dry the hair smooth.

Step 2 Section out a channel of hair with a tail comb to create the direction of the design required.

Step 3 Use a sectioning clip to secure the other parts of the remainder hair out of the way.

Remember

 Regardless of whether you are doing scalp plaits, singles or twists, the direction in which they flow is related to their starting position on the scalp. Your accurate sectioning creates this.

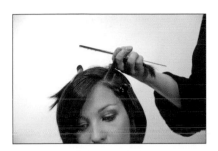

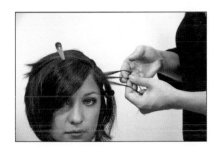

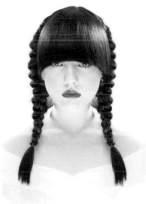

Step 4 For cane rows without added hair, subdivide the client's hair from the front of the channelled section into 3 stems.

Step 5 Holding the front, first section between the middle and third finger of the left hand and the next, middle section between the index finger and thumb. Now take the last or third section, between the middle and third finger of the right hand.

Step 6 Pass the middle section with the index finger of the left hand under the last outer section of the right hand and pass the new middle section under the outer section of the left hand.

Step 7 Pick up a little hair along the channel with the fourth finger and incorporate into the outer third stem.

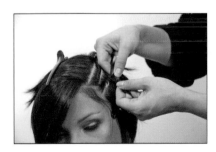

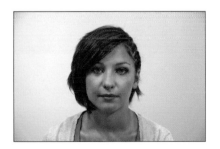

Step 8 Repeat steps 6 and 7 until you have worked along the complete channel of hair until the point where the plait leaves the scalp to hang freely, then continue plaiting the single, three stems until all of the hair is plaited.

Step 9 Secure the ends with a covered professional band and start steps 2–9 again on the next cane row.

Applying twisting techniques

Twists are an alternative to plaited styles; they will last for up to a month before they become untidy. Unlike plaits, they don't involve any interlocking of hair, so they usually require an application of pomade or light styling gel to bond the hair while the twists are being formed.

Twisting uses the fingers or a comb to twist the hair into strands. This can be done in linear patterns along the scalp such as flat twists, or off the scalp as with single twists or 2-stem twists.

Step by step: flat twist

The flat twist has a similar appearance, at a distance, to cornrows, but when you look more closely you can see that the hair isn't interlocked in the same way. The durability of the effects depends upon the type of hair, but as a rule of thumb, twists don't last as long as cornrows. However, they don't take anything like the same amount of time to put in as tight, 3-stem scalp plaits.

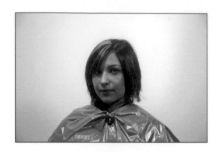

Step 1 Shampoo (and condition if necessary) and dry the hair roughly into shape.

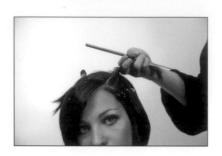

Step 2 After brushing the hair to remove any tangles, start at the front by dividing the hair into a single channel about 1 cm wide.

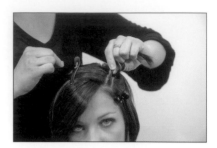

Step 3 Start twisting from the front, back towards the crown area, making sure that the twists are comfortable and not too tight.

Step 4 Secure the end of the completed twist with a grip.

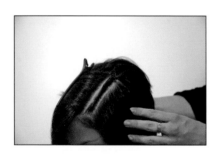

Step 5 Continue by starting another twist next to and parallel to the first one in exactly the same way.

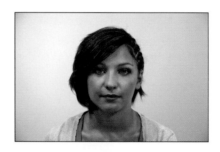

Step 6 Complete each twist in sequence until you have worked around the head.

Step 7 The remaining hair can then be dressed in either a casual or formal effect.

Step-by-step 2-stem twists

Step 1 Shampoo (and condition if necessary) and towel dry the hair.

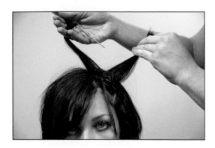

Step 2 Divide the hair into 4 quadrants and secure with sectioning clips.

Step 3 Section off horizontally at the nape and secure the remainder out of the way. Subdivide the horizontal sections into smaller areas of just a few millimetres across. (The smaller the sections the tidier the twist will look.)

Step 4 Apply the gel or pomade throughout the length of the twist stem.

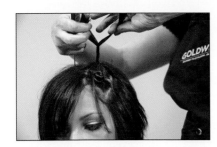

Step 5 Subdivide the single stem, making 2 stems and start twisting left over right (or vice versa).

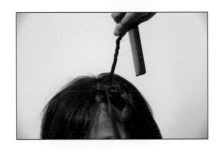

Step 6 Continue through the length of the hair.

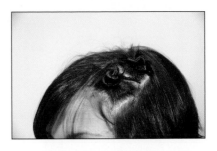

Step 7 Continue on to the next twist in the horizontal section and repeat steps 5 and 6. Continue working up the head.

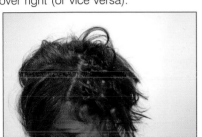

Step 8 When all of the twists have been completed, arrange them neatly in the direction of the desired style and place under a dryer for 20–30 minutes. When completely dry, apply product – either a spray fixative or sheen – to complete the look.

Remember

 If hair is left in a plaited or twisted style for too long, the quality and condition of the hair can deteriorate. Potential effects include:

● dryness and brittleness – the hair lacks moisture
● hair damage or breakage
● traction alopecia from constant root tension
● hair knotting or matted and impossible to remove without cutting
● scalp dryness and flaking.

Senegalese twists

Senegalese twists are a scalp twist effect; they consist of stems of hair that are always twisted in the same direction with hair crossing over and creating a rope effect. This is the method:

1 Shampoo (condition if necessary) and pre-dry the hair smooth.

2 Section out a channel of hair with a tail comb to create the direction and the design required.

3 Using the fingers, start close to the root, take a small section of hair and twist it in a clockwise movement.

4 As you work along the channel, pick up and work in more sections of hair to create the scalp twist effect.

5 When the channel of twisted hair is finished, secure until all of the others are finished.

6 The free ends of the twists can be interlocked together, and then after they have been dried under a dryer the effect can be thermally styled to complete the total effect.

Checkerboard

	I know and understand the health, safety and hygiene aspects of plaiting and twisting hair ☐	I know how to prepare the client, tools and the work area correctly ☐	I can recognise the signs of traction alopecia and know what causes it ☐
I know how to minimise the risk of cross-infection and cross-infestation ☐	I know the ranges of products available and how they should be used on the hair ☐	I know how to create a range of plaiting and twisted effects on short, medium and longer hair ☐	I always follow the instructions given to me by the stylist and I always follow the manufacturer's instructions when using materials ☐
I know how to secure plaits and twists with professional bands ☐	I always check that the client is comfortable throughout the service ☐	I know the problems associated with plaiting and twisting and what care I should take ☐	

Revision questions

Q1 Fill in the blank: _____ alopecia is a condition caused by excessive tension upon the hair.

Q2 Cornrows are also known as cane rows. True or false?

Q3 Which of the following techniques would take less than 30 minutes to complete? (You may choose more than one answer.)

1	a French plait	4	a full head of scalp twists
2	a full head of cornrows	5	a full head of cane rows
3	a "pony" tail	6	a full head of twisted knots

Q4 Cornrows is a close "head hugging" design made up of several scalp plaits. True or false?

Q5 Which of the following is the odd one out? (Choose one answer.)

a	cornrows	c	Senegalese twists
b	cane rows	d	French plait

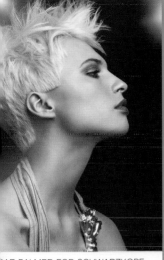

RAE PALMER FOR SCHWARZKOPF,
PHOTOGRAPHY:
ANDREW O'TOOLE **GH7**

GH7.1

GH7.2

**CREDIT VALUE
FOR UNIT GH7**
3 Credits

Unit title

GH7 Remove hair
extensions

This is an **optional** unit for
Level 1. It is made up of 2
main outcomes.

Main outcomes

GH7 (eku1) Maintain effective and safe methods of
working when removing hair
extensions

GH7 (eku2) Remove hair
extensions

Chapter**ten**
Remove hair extensions

Unit GH7: quick overview

What do I need to do for GH7.1?

You need to **prepare for removing extensions** by:

- correctly protect and position clients and yourself
- keeping work areas clean at all times
- maintaining personal hygiene standards
- using tools and materials safely

What do I need to do for GH7.2?

You need to **remove extensions** by:

- listening to the stylist's instructions
- minimising the risk of hair damage
- ensuring that the client is comfortable
- preparing the hair for the service
- learning about removal techniques

What things do I need to cover?

You will be removing:

- hot and cold bonded extensions

Using:

- seam releasers
- scissors
- seal breakers
- chemical solutions

Keywords

Cold-fusion hair extensions
a system of connecting hair extensions by using adhesives and adhesive strips

Cornrows
(also known as cane rows) a term used to describe an effect created by multiple rows of plaits that follow the contour of the head

Hot-bonded hair extensions
a system of connecting hair extensions by using resin or hard plastics

Removal solution
a chemical formulated to dissolve the adhesive connecting the hair extension to the hair in cold-fusion systems

Removal tool
a metal pair of pliers used for breaking the bond connecting the hair extension to the hair in hot-bonded systems

Traction alopecia
a condition that is caused by the excessive pulling of hair at the root, it is often associated with longer hair worn in plaits, twists, hair-ups and extensions

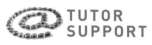 **TUTOR SUPPORT**

Task 10.1 Process of adding the extensions to the hair and how they are removed

What things do I need to know?

You need to **know and understand**:

- your salon's way of preparing and protecting the clients
- your salon's procedures for the disposal of waste items
- your salon's service timings
- what contact dermatitis is and how to avoid developing it
- how to clean and prepare the salon's work areas
- how to work safely and hygienically at all times
- how to use and maintain the removal tools
- how to reassure clients experiencing concern or anxiety during the process
- the average rate of hair growth
- the consequences of excess tension on hair and the indicators of traction alopecia
- why extensions should be removed in a recommended timeframe
- the ways in which hair extensions are removed

Introduction

Hair extensions are a popular alternative for clients that want instant changes.

Hair extensions give clients an instant, exciting new image

The range of hair extension systems available allows clients to have either a temporary effect for a special occasion or longer lasting looks that they can wear for several months. You will be learning how to assist the stylist by removing the different types of hair extension in preparation for partial and total replacement services. Before looking at the particular techniques for removing hair extensions, it may be worthwhile looking at the range of hair extension systems that are available and the range of looks that they can achieve.

Hair extension systems

There are 4 main hair extension systems that are used to apply strands or wefts of extension hair into a client's hairstyle:

- **hot-bonded hair extensions**
- **cold-fusion hair extensions**
- plaited/braided extensions
- sewn-in extensions.

Each of these systems has a particular way in which the extensions should be removed, and you will need to be familiar with all the techniques.

Hot-bonded extension system   This is the most popular and widely used extension system in the UK. Heated tools are used to melt a polymer resin, creating a hard bond that attaches the extensions near the root area of the client's natural hair. It is suitable for all hair types except African Caribbean hair and allows the stylist to apply individual extension strands to create freely flowing hairstyles that move like real hair. This system uses a removal tool, similar to a pair of pliers, to break the seals and remove the extension from the hair. The hair can then be prepared for further services.

Cold-fusion extension system   This type of system uses adhesives, solutions or tapes to hold strands or wefts of extension hair in place on natural hair. Cold-fusion systems create bonds that can be used on any hair type. Regardless of method used, they are removed by the careful application of a chemical bond removing solution.

Plaited/braided extensions   This method uses plaiting techniques to add extension hair into a hairstyle. This does not produce a freely flowing hairstyle but can be applied to many hair lengths and types. They can be released by carefully cutting them out of the client's natural hair.

Sewn-in extensions   This is a popular system for applying wefts of natural or synthetic fibre extensions on to pre-plaited scalp braids called **cornrows**. The wefts are sewn onto the braids using a curved needle and thread. They are particularly popular on African Caribbean hair and other curly hair types. Removal involves great care as, like plaits and braids, they are cut to release them from the client's natural hair.

Hair extension hairstyles

The types of hairstyles that can be created by hair extensions fall into four categories:

- hair additions
- hair enhancements
- hair extensions
- hair alternatives

Hair additions are applied to the client's natural hair as strands to give subtle or vibrant contrasts to their own colour, for example, as highlights, lowlights, colour flashes and slices. This system provides an alternative to permanent colouring and adds more fibre or hair to the client's original hair, making the hair thicker than before. This is particularly useful if the client has fine hair.

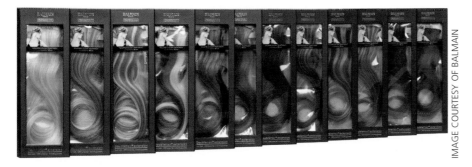

Hair additions come in a variety of colours

Hair enhancements are applied as strands, or more popularly as rows of wefts. They will thicken the client's natural hair, giving more body and make the natural hair look longer. They are quick to apply, available in a wide range of natural and synthetic hair colours and lengths, and reusable if they are looked after and maintained.

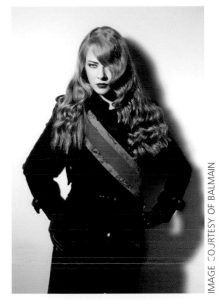

IMAGE COURTESY OF BALMAIN

Extensions can give a natural, lush look

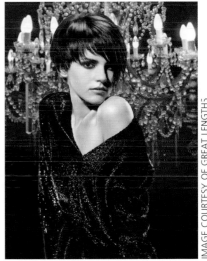

IMAGE COURTESY OF GREAT LENGTHS

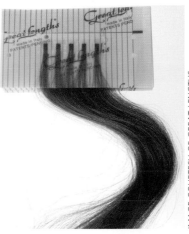

IMAGE COURTESY OF GREAT LENGTHS

Hair enhancements make the natural hair look longer

IMAGE COURTESY OF BALMAIN

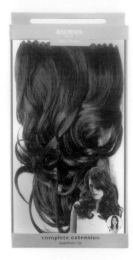

Hair extensions are individual strand extensions

Remember

After three months, the remaining original extensions are so far away from the scalp that they must all be removed, even if only to be replaced with new hair extensions.

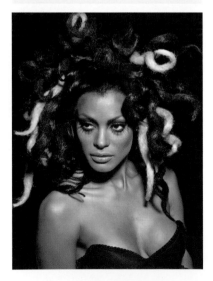

Hair alternatives are bold and avant-garde

EKU *statement*

GH7 (eku20) the average rate of hair growth

GH7 (eku23) how wearing extensions beyond their recommended time period can affect the removal process

Hair extensions are applied using 150–250 individual strand extensions that can be either pre-bonded natural hair or synthetic fibre. The colours can be matched to the client's own hair, giving natural effects, can be multi-toned as highlights or lowlights, or blended to give a variety of fashion effects. These give clients an immediate, longer, free flowing hairstyle.

Hair alternatives are a texture fibre or real extension made by the stylist into a braid, a twisted effect like a dreadlock, or any unnaturally occurring effect. Because of this, the styles are more exaggerated or avant-garde in their appearance and will only suit those people with the confidence to wear them.

Maintenance

Hair extensions do not last forever. Even if they are applied to the root area using a hot-bonded system, they will gradually grow out. Hair grows at an average rate of 1.25 cm per month, so within a couple of months the extensions could be more than 2.5 cm away from the scalp. But even before this, because of general wear and tear, many of these will need replacing to "tidy up".

Maintenance appointments for hair extensions are an essential part of the complete service. When the stylist initially consults with the client, they will be looking for an ongoing commitment in maintaining the look. This means that the client will book their "tidy up" appointment around 4–6 weeks after the original extension service. During this appointment, the stylist will select the extensions that need to be replaced. You will be removing these so that the hair is prepared for the re-application of new extensions in this area.

Remember

People naturally lose 80 to 100 hairs per day; these are normally replaced at the same rate with new hair so we don't end up prematurely bald. However, for clients with hair extensions, this "hair fall" creates another problem. As the hair grows and falls away from the scalp, it can't fall away from the hairstyle because it is bonded to the extensions. Within three months this looks very "fluffy" or "fuzzy" because the entwined hair will tangle and the frizziness can't be combed away. Some bonds can leave tiny knots in the natural hair around the root area that can be very difficult to comb out.

The complete head of extensions need to be removed during the removal appointment, so that the hair can be re-conditioned and made ready for further extensions or other services. The removal appointment is the final hair extension maintenance appointment, which is booked 12 weeks after the original hair extensions were applied.

Removal

The length of time booked for the removal of extensions during the maintenance appointment will depend on the bonding system used. For example, a full head of extensions applied by a hot-bonded system can take up to 3 hours. A partial head replacement of extensions for the same system can take up to an hour or so to remove. However, the removal of sewn-in extensions may take considerably less time because complete wefts of hair are quicker to remove than strands. When the thread is cut, the whole weft is released, leaving the natural hair in its braided scalp plaits effect.

Activity
Preparing for hair extension removal
Complete this activity by filling in the missing information in the table below.

Preparation	What do you need to do?
client	
yourself	
tools/materials	

GH7.1 Maintain effective and safe methods of working when removing hair extensions

The general aspects of working safely are covered in Chapter 1, Make sure your own actions reduce risks to health and safety, pages 12 to 19. Please review this chapter for more information.

Correctly protect and position clients and yourself

Make sure that the client is adequately protected throughout the service. They should be wearing a full gown and towel, and possibly a cape too, so that they are protected from falling hair clippings, hard seal fragments and spills from removal solutions.

A full head of hair extensions, even temporary ones, takes a long time to apply and the removal can be equally as long. So the main health and safety concerns relate to the

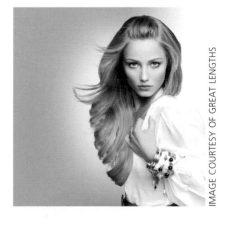

Remember

The removal of hair extensions takes a long time. This is true even just for a "tidy up" appointment, and you will be standing throughout the process. Take particular care with your standing position and your posture. See Chapter 1, Make sure your own actions reduce risks to health and safety, in the section on personal wellbeing on page 21.

length of time that you will be standing whilst doing the work, and the client's comfort, positioning and protection during the process.

In addition to your posture and positioning, you must take every care in the way that you handle and use the equipment because:

- it is easy to spill removal chemicals on the client
- you may be using removal equipment that could easily slip and injure yourself or the client, or damage their hair
- you will need to keep an even tension on the client's hair whilst you work, without putting too much pressure on their hair or scalp.

Specific risks associated with hair extension services

There are some specific risks associated with hair extension services. These are outlined below.

You must	... because there is a risk that
Keep your nails trimmed, and hands and jewellery clean	... you might pass on infections with dirty hands, nails or jewellery.
Keep jewellery on your hands or around your wrists to a minimum	... if jewellery gets caught in the extensions they may need cutting out to remove them.
Wear comfortable, loose-fitting clothes and shoes	... you will tire and feel uncomfortable very quickly as you will be standing for a long period.
Make sure that your client is sitting in a height-adjustable chair	... you will get back ache, neck ache or fatigue if you work in the wrong position.
Sterilise the tools that you will be using on the client	... you could cross-infect the client by using unhygienic tools.
Work in a well-ventilated area when you use removal solutions	... you or the client could become ill from the vapours these products give off.
Clear up any chemical spills immediately	... the floor will become slippery and a hazard to everyone. ... if these spill on to the client it could damage their clothes.
Wear disposable vinyl gloves when handling removal solutions	... these products could cause contact dermatitis – see Chapter 1 for more information.

EKU statement

GH7 (eku5) what is contact dermatitis and how to avoid developing it whilst carrying out hair attachment services

Remember

Always wear the PPE (disposable gloves and plastic apron) provided by your salon when carrying out technical services.

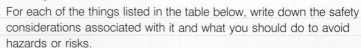

Activity

For each of the things listed in the table below, write down the safety considerations associated with it and what you should do to avoid hazards or risks.

Area of work	Safety consideration	What should you do to avoid hazards or risks?
cold-fusion systems		
hot-bonded systems		
standing during the removal process		
keeping the work area tidy		

Keeping work areas clean at all times

The environment that you work in whilst performing the removal service must be perfectly clean. Workstations, hairdressing trolleys, any work surfaces and surrounding floor areas must be kept spotless. Keep cotton wool swabs and cloths close at hand so that you can quickly attend to any chemical spills on the client or the floor.

Maintaining personal hygiene standards

All the materials that come into contact with the client's skin must be clean and hygienic. Similarly, your own personal standards of health and hygiene should not present any risk to the client either. This will prevent the risk of cross-infection and helps to maintain a healthy, safe environment.

For more information on preventing infection and personal health and hygiene, see Chapter 1, Make sure your own actions reduce risks to health and safety, pages 14–15 and 20.

> **Activity**
>
> Write the answers to the following questions in your portfolio.
>
> 1 Why is it important to keep the work area clean and tidy?
>
> 2 How is the risk of cross-infection minimised?
>
> 3 How should you stand when removing hair extensions?
>
> 4 When should you wear PPE and why?
>
> 5 How would you know if a client is comfortable or not?

Using tools and materials safely

You will be handling and using many of the tools and materials that the stylists do in their work, so you must be familiar with how they are used safely and correctly.

Synthetic (artificial) fibre extension hair

Synthetic, or artificial, extension hair is made of a man-made fibre that is specifically designed to create hair extension hairstyles. It is pre-coloured in a wide range of tones and is prepared to provide the following textures:

- straight lengths in strands or wefts
- wavy lengths as wefts
- curly lengths as wefts
- ringlets as wefts
- plaits as wefts
- dreadlocks as wefts.

Artificial hair can feel, look and move like hair in great condition. It is made from acrylic, however, which is particularly sensitive to heat. It is very easy to damage or ruin its

EKU *statement*

GH7 (eku12) why it is important to keep your work area clean and tidy

GH7 (eku13) methods of cleaning, disinfecting and/ or sterilisation used in salons

GH7 (eku14) methods of working safely and hygienically and which minimise the risk of cross-infection and cross-infestation

EKU *statement*

GH7 (eku16) the importance of personal hygiene

EKU *statement*

GH7 (eku26) the types of products to use when removing hot and cold hair extension systems.

GH7 (eku15) the correct use and maintenance of removal tools

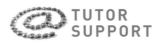

TUTOR SUPPORT

Task 10.2 Effects hair extension hairstyles can create

Remember

Hair extensions are pre-processed to create different structures. This refers to the physical appearance of the hair extension, which can be strands, ringlets, plaits or dreadlocks.

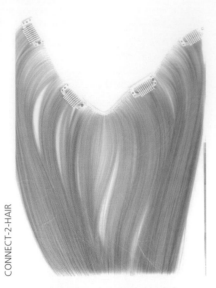

A synthetic fibre extension weft

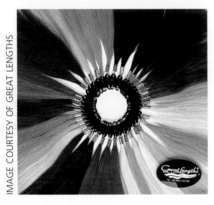

Extensions made of real hair usually come from the Far East or Eastern Europe

Remember

Real hair extensions must always lie with natural hair in the same root to point direction to avoid tangling and matting.

EKU *statement*

GH7 (eku19) the importance of checking you have understood the instructions given by the stylist

qualities if the fibre is brought into contact with heat or heated equipment. The client will have been made aware of this at the time when the extensions were first applied. You must take care when handling this material so that you don't degrade the quality of the fibre. The stylist would also have taken a lot of care in handling the fibres when they were first applied. The extension wefts would have been kept flat and smooth so that they didn't tangle or knot before they were applied. You should take care when handling the material to avoid tangling and knotting too.

Real extension hair

Real hair extensions are Asian or European in origin. They have been prepared by cleansing in caustic soda (which removes any infestation) and then coloured, lightened or permed to create the required structure. During this processing, the lengths of hair have to be kept in the same root to point direction. This has to be followed through during application as well, otherwise the hair will matt or lock together. This matting occurs because if the hair's natural cuticle layer lies together in different directions, the hair tangles and becomes impossible to maintain. Real hair can be bonded together as sewn wefts, bulk lengths or pre-bonded lengths. The weft looks like a curtain of hair. It can be made up into narrow or wide lengths, with the root end being bonded by machine or hand stitching. Take care when handling the material to avoid tangling as tangled hair cannot be used and is wasteful.

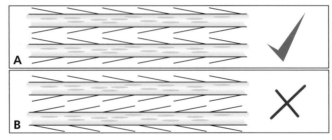

Hair lying (A) cuticle edges in same direction, and (B) cuticle edges in opposite directions

Removal solutions

These chemical products are formulated by the manufacturers to work with cold-fusion systems and are applied directly to the bonds to dissolve the adhesive and release the hair extension from the client's natural hair. They are acetone or alcohol based and must always be used following the manufacturer's instructions. They are patented products that are matched to specific cold-fusion systems; it is essential that the correct removal solution be used.

Removal tools

Removal tools are metal instruments that look like pliers; they are designed to crush the adhesive bond that holds the extension in place for hot-bonded systems. You must take care when using them because it is very easy to pull or damage the client's hair whilst removing their extensions. They can be sterilised in the same way that other metal tools are cleaned and maintained in an autoclave or UV cabinet. See the section on sterilisation in Chapter 1, Make sure your own actions reduce risks to health and safety, page 15, for more information.

Listening to the stylist's instructions

The stylist will have consulted the client and decided on the correct course of action. This will be either:

- the removal of selected hair extensions that have grown away from the root area and now need replacing, or
- the removal of all the extensions so that the hair is prepared for further services.

You will be working under the close supervision of the stylist; you must follow their instructions. Only remove the extensions that they have specified, follow the removal method that they specify and only use the tools and materials that they tell you to.

Minimising the risk of hair damage

Traction alopecia

One of the more serious after effects of wearing hair extensions is **traction alopecia**. This occurs when a constant pressure, such as wearing hair tied up or weight from hair extensions, is exerted upon the roots of the hair. It can result in hair loss in patches upon the scalp (baldness), and is particularly obvious in areas of weaker hair such as the temples or hairlines.

If the client tells you that they have had unpleasant tightness in any area since the extensions were applied, you should tell the stylist immediately because this may affect the removal process. Similarly, if you find sore or thinning areas on the scalp, tell the stylist immediately.

Ensuring that the client is comfortable

Removing extensions takes a long time, even for a "tidy up" appointment, and the client will be seated in the same position throughout. Stop now and again to give both you and the client a bit of a break. You could always offer to make them a drink, or they might need to pop to the toilet.

It's often difficult to hold a conversation whilst you are concentrating on what you are doing. (Don't worry – many stylists have the same problem; even with several years of experience!) However, long periods of silence can be uncomfortable, particularly when the client doesn't understand what is going on. Try to be reassuring. People tend to get edgy when they wait for a long time and very little (as far as they are concerned) seems to be happening. Make a point of explaining what you are doing now and then. This keeps them informed and this prevents their boredom turning into panic!

The client will sense your level of confidence. If you show signs of anxiety, the client will get stressed too. If they then start to panic, you will naturally sense it too and it "winds up" the stress level. Keep calm; if you find that a particular area or bond is difficult to remove; take your time. It will work eventually (you can always call the stylist for help).

Remember

If you are not sure what has been asked of you, ask the stylist to explain again.

EKU statement

GH7 (eku22) how to identify the signs of traction alopecia

GH7 (eku21) the potential consequences of excessive tension on the hair

EKU statement

GH7 (eku17) the types of anxieties commonly experienced by clients undergoing the hair extension removal process

GH7 (eku18) how to give reassurance to clients

Remember

Taking a pair of pliers to someone's hair can look frightening! Explain what you are doing, why you are doing it and roughly how long it will take.

Remember

Simple words of reassurance reduce panic and remove stress. Keep things light-hearted: humour is a great way to break down barriers. Reassurance can run along the lines of saying things like, "Yes, this is normal – it often takes a bit longer to get Steve's extensions out. He puts them in so well."

Activity

This activity considers how the client might be feeling throughout the removal process. Look at the table below and write down your answers in each of the following situations.

Situation	What signs would they be showing?	What would you do?
the client feels anxious about what you are doing		
the client is worried about their hair extensions		
the client is feeling uncomfortable		

Activity

Write down your answers to the following questions in your portfolio.

1 What are the signs of traction alopecia?

2 What is the average rate of growth of hair?

3 Why shouldn't a client wear hair extensions for more than 3 months?

4 What is the difference between a cold-fusion system and a hot-bonded system?

5 What is the difference between a hair addition and a hair alternative?

6 Which way should natural hair extensions lie in relation to a client's own hair?

EKU *statement*

GH7 (eku24) how to remove hot and cold hair extension systems

GH7 (eku25) the generally accepted sequence of working for removing hair extensions

Remember

Always check that you are using the correct removal solution for the right cold-fusion system.

TUTOR SUPPORT

Task 10.4 How long each of the extension methods should be left in the hair

Preparing the hair for the service

If the stylist is going to reapply the hair extensions on the same day as the removal, you will need to shampoo the natural hair with a clarifying shampoo prior to the reapplication. This will remove any traces of conditioner or product build-up. Build-up may affect the effectiveness of the bonding of the newly applied extensions. Dry the hair into style and brush well to remove any loose hairs. See Chapter 5, Shampoo and condition hair.

Learning about removal techniques

Gather all the things that you need on your trolley. This may include:

- the correct removal solution
- cotton wool pads
- disposable vinyl gloves
- removal tool
- an old pair of hairdressing scissors
- hair clips
- comb and soft bristle brush.

Cold-fusion adhesive tape strip removal

Self-adhesive extensions need a special chemical spray or solution to dissolve the bond attaching them to the hair, so put on your gloves and apron before doing anything. When the removal solution is applied/sprayed onto the self-cling tape strip, it quickly reduces the adhesion and therefore releases the weft from the hair. The removed weft can then be inspected to see if it is worth keeping or whether it should be thrown away.

The self-cling strips can be removed from the weft in the same way that the extension is removed from the hair. Depending on the quality of the weft, it can be washed, re-conditioned and retained for future use, or otherwise disposed of. If the weft is to be re-used, new, double-sided self-adhesive tape strips will need to be applied after the wefts have been dried.

Remember

 Always detangle the hair and brush it through after you remove each hair extension.

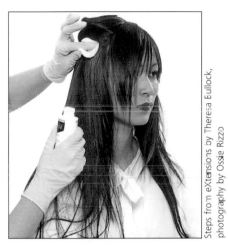

Steps from eXtensions by Theresa Bullock, photography by Ossie Rizzo

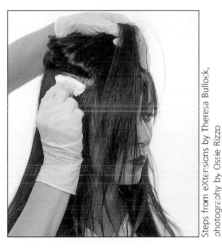

Steps from eXtensions by Theresa Bullock, photography by Ossie Rizzo

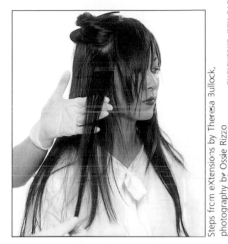

Steps from eXtensions by Theresa Bullock, photography by Ossie Rizzo

Step 1 Pour a small amount of the removal solution onto a cottonwool pad. Wipe the top side of the tape near the root area then lift the tape weft and wipe the underside of the weft.

Step 2 Allow the removal solution to penetrate for 30 seconds to one minute.

Step 3 Hold the end of the extension hair contained in the tape and gently pull it away from the hair and scalp. The weft comes away easily from the natural hair in a matter of seconds.

Cold-fusion bonded weft removal

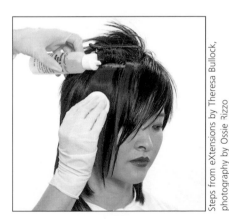

Steps from eXtensions by Theresa Bullock, photography by Ossie Rizzo

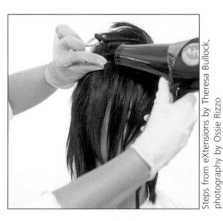

Steps from eXtensions by Theresa Bullock, photography by Ossie Rizzo

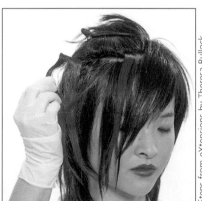

Steps from eXtensions by Theresa Bullock, photography by Ossie Rizzo

Step 1 Place a cotton wool pad next to the scalp underneath the weft of extension hair. Apply the removal solution for this system directly onto the weft of extension hair; the cotton wool will catch drips. Using the dampened cotton wool pad, wipe the solution evenly across the weft, leave the solution to penetrate through the weft and onto the natural hair for one minute.

Step 2 Using a hairdryer heat the weft at the root area for three minutes. Heat activates the removal solution, breaking down the cold-fusion adhesive.

Step 3 Once the adhesive is softened the weft is ready to peel off. Remove the weft carefully, reapplying removal solution where applicable.

Hot-bond strand removal with removal tool and solution

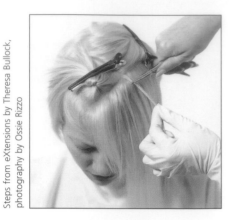

Steps from eXtensions by Theresa Bullock, photography by Ossie Rizzo

Step 1 Take a removal tool and crush along the length of the bond.

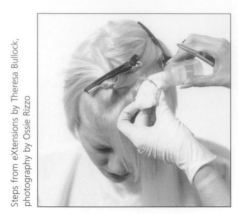

Steps from eXtensions by Theresa Bullock, photography by Ossie Rizzo

Step 2 Place a cottonwool pad underneath the bond, to catch any drips of solution. Apply removal solution to the bond fold the cottonwool pad over the bond and hold it for 1–3 minutes; this allows the solution to penetrate the bond.

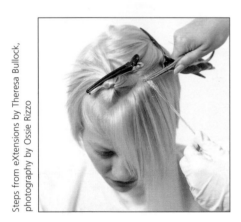

Steps from eXtensions by Theresa Bullock, photography by Ossie Rizzo

Step 3 Crush the bond using the removal tool.

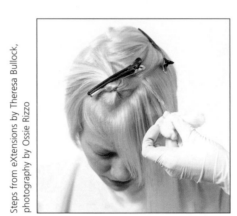

Steps from eXtensions by Theresa Bullock, photography by Ossie Rizzo

Step 4 As the bonds crumbles and breaks down pull the extension hair gently away from the natural hair.

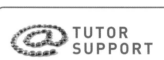

TUTOR SUPPORT

Task 10.5 PPE for removing extensions and how the client should be protected

Hot-bond strand removal with removal solution

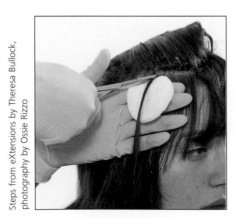

Steps from eXtensions by Theresa Bullock, photography by Ossie Rizzo

Step 1 Place a cotton wool pad underneath the extension bond. Apply the removal solution for this resin.

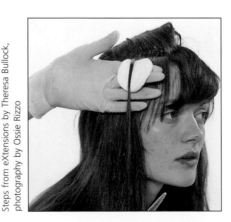

Steps from eXtensions by Theresa Bullock, photography by Ossie Rizzo

Step 2 Keeping the pad in place, apply pressure to either side of the bond with a removal tool. The bond is broken in three places: at the top, middle and bottom.

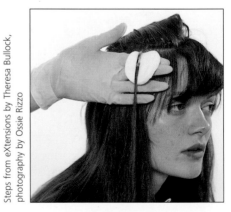

Steps from eXtensions by Theresa Bullock, photography by Ossie Rizzo

Step 3 Holding the natural hair at the root, pull the extension strand at the end point for a clean removal.

Sewn wefts removal

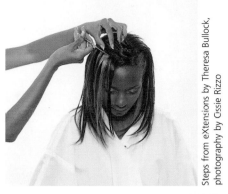

Steps from *Extensions* by Theresa Bullock, photography by Ossie Rizzo

Using old hairdressing scissors carefully cut the stitches that hold the weft in place. The weft will fall from the natural hair.

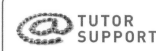

TUTOR SUPPORT

Task 10.3 Types of hair extensions

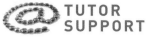

TUTOR SUPPORT

Task 10.6 Health and safety when removing extensions

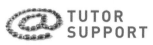

TUTOR SUPPORT

Short answer tests

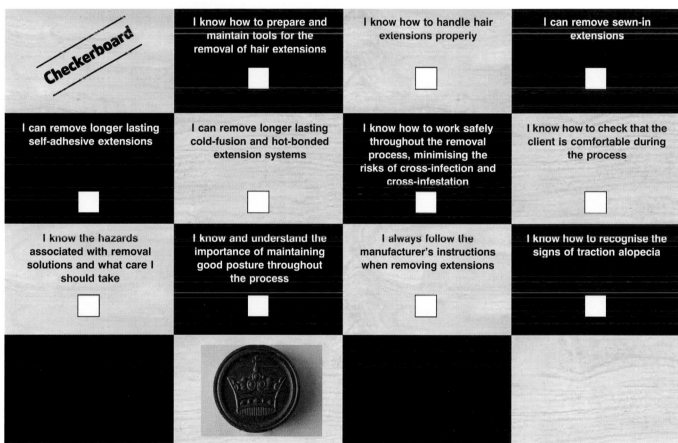

Checkerboard	I know how to prepare and maintain tools for the removal of hair extensions ☐	I know how to handle hair extensions properly ☐	I can remove sewn-in extensions ☐
I can remove longer lasting self-adhesive extensions ☐	I can remove longer lasting cold-fusion and hot-bonded extension systems ☐	I know how to work safely throughout the removal process, minimising the risks of cross-infection and cross-infestation ☐	I know how to check that the client is comfortable during the process ☐
I know the hazards associated with removal solutions and what care I should take ☐	I know and understand the importance of maintaining good posture throughout the process ☐	I always follow the manufacturer's instructions when removing extensions ☐	I know how to recognise the signs of traction alopecia ☐

Revision questions

Q1 Fill in the blank: A removal solution is a chemical formulated to —— the adhesive connecting the hair extension to the hair.

Q2 Cold-fusion hair extensions are a system of connecting hair extensions by using heated resin. True or false?

Q3 What are the 4 main techniques for bonding extensions to hair? (Choose 4 answers.)

1	grafting	**3**	cold-fusion	**5**	plaiting
2	hot-bonded	**4**	sewing	**6**	twisting

Q4 Cold-fusion systems use adhesives, solutions or tapes to hold strands or wefts of extension hair in place on natural hair. True or false?

Q5 A removal tool is used for which type of hair extensions? (Choose one answer.)

a	cold-fusion systems	**c**	clip-on wefts
b	hot-bonded systems	**d**	self-adhesive strands

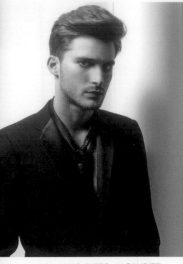

Chapter**eleven**
Assist with shaving services

GB1

GB1.1

GB1.2

CREDIT VALUE FOR UNIT GB1

2 Credits

Unit title

GB1 Assist with shaving services

This is an **optional** unit for Level 1. It is made up of 2 main outcomes.

Main outcomes

GB1 (eku1) Maintain effective and safe methods of working when assisting with shaving services

GB1 (eku2) Prepare facial hair and skin for shaving services

Unit GB1: quick overview

What do I need to do for GB1.1?

You need to **assist in the preparation for shaving** by:

- correctly protect and position clients and yourself
- keeping work areas clean and safe to use at all times
- maintaining personal hygiene standards
- cleaning tools and equipment
- dealing with waste and shortages
- learning about shaving products

What do I need to do for GB1.2?

You need to **assist in the shaving process** by:

- cleansing and exfoliating the skin
- applying hot and cold towels
- applying lathering products
- telling the barber when the client is prepared
- removing lather and cooling the skin

What things do I need to cover?

You will using:

- creams and oils

Applied by:

- brushes and massage techniques

What things do I need to know?

You need to **know and understand**:

- your salon's way of preparing and protecting the clients
- how to work safely and hygienically at all times
- what contact dermatitis is and how to avoid developing it
- how to sterilise and prepare the tools and equipment
- how to prepare towels and lathering products and what effects they have
- how and when to use brushes or massage techniques for applying the lather
- how to remove the lathering products

Introduction

The purpose of shaving is to remove unwanted hair, and most men consider this to be a daily chore; a routine that should be carried out as quickly as possible, so that they can get on with their busy lives. However, it needn't be, as the barber has made this a relaxing and luxuriant service that you will be helping to provide.

Shaving need not be a chore!

The barber's shave

The everyday routine of shaving for many men is a tedious necessity; it takes up extra time in a busy lifestyle. The barber's shave is considered to be a luxury, but still a valuable service.

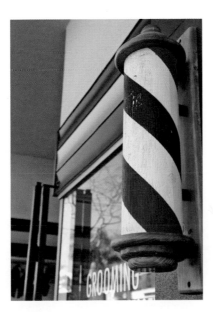

The barber's pole

Keywords

Body odour
(BO) the result of poor personal hygiene and lack of regular washing

Dermatitis
an occupational disease that affects the skin causing an itching sensation accompanied by reddening and dry cracked areas

Effleurage
a light stroking movement applied with either the fingers or the palms of the hands

Exfoliate
to scrub skin with a gritty substance to remove the dead cells of the surface layer

Halitosis
bad breath

Moisturising balms
cooling, soothing and moisture replenishing lotions applied after shaving to counteract the abrasive effects of the process

Petrissage
a kneading movement of the skin that lifts and compresses underlying structures of the skin

Sharps box
a designated sealed container used for the safe disposal of sharp items, e.g. used razor blades

GB1.1   Maintain effective and safe methods of working when assisting with shaving services

EKU *statements*

GB1 (eku1) your salon's requirements for client preparation

GB1 (eku5) what is contact dermatitis and how to avoid developing it whilst assisting with shaving services

GB1 (eku6) the range of protective equipment that should be available for clients

GB1 (eku7) the type of personal protective equipment available

GB1 (eku8) why it is important to use personal protective equipment

GB1 (eku9) how the position of your client and yourself can affect the desired outcome and reduce fatigue and the risk of injury

GB1 (eku11) the importance of using the correct type of barber's chair for shaving services

You will be using a range of shaving equipment and products. These materials need to be handled safely and made hygienically clean so that they are ready for use. This includes the sterilisation of brushes, bowls etc. See Cleaning the tools and equipment after they have been used, pages 148–50, for more information.

Correctly protect and position clients and yourself

Gowning the client

Always use fresh, clean, laundered equipment. This is the gowning procedure:

- fasten a gown at the back, or secure the cutting square with a clip to ensure that the covering is close fitting around the neck and protects the client from any spillages
- place a towel around the front of the client so that the free edges are fastened at the back
- tuck a strip of neck wool (or neck tissue) in to the top edge of the towel to stop lather and hair fragments from falling inside the client's clothes.

Positioning the client

Client posture The client sits with their head tilted back. You need to work at an angle that enables you to work safely and carefully. If you need to recline the chair, do it before the client is seated. Ensure that the client is seated all the way back in the chair with their feet squarely on the footrests.

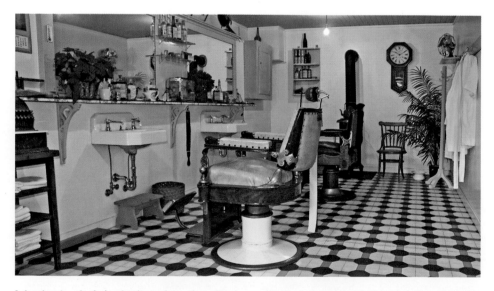

A barber's chair is designed so the client can tilt their head back for shaving services

The client's posture should:

- prevent them from twisting or "hunching up"
- allow them to sit with the head supported for long periods of time in a position that doesn't give them any discomfort or risk of injury or fatigue
- give you the access and freedom to work on the client properly and safely.

Ask the client if they are comfortable, and if you need to make any adjustments to working height or angle, do it before proceeding with the service.

Your working posture Barbering involves a lot of standing, and because of this you will need to be comfortable in your work. You should always adopt a comfortable but safe work position. Sometimes comfortable and safe are not necessarily the same thing. A naturally comfortable position for work should allow you to:

- stand close enough to the styling chair without touching it
- position your shoulders and torso directly above your hips and feet, with your weight evenly distributed
- not have to twist at any point, so you can easily work around the chair or get your client to turn their head slightly towards you
- wear comfortable shoes, so that your body weight is comfortably supported on the widest parts of the feet, which will allow you to work for longer periods of time without risk to injury or fatigue.

Lift your arms to check the working height. If you have to raise your arms anywhere near horizontal during your work, you will find that they will start to ache very quickly. Make your adjustments to the styling chair, either up or down to suit your needs. Don't forget to tell the client before you adjust the chair – it might be a little shocking when they find themselves being "jacked" up to the ceiling!

Shaving position The client's shaving position and height from the floor have a direct effect on your working position. You must be able to work in a position where everything that you will need is at hand; you should be able to access the hot towels, lathering products and equipment easily. Follow these procedures:

1 Adjust the seated client's chair height to a position where you can work upright without having to over-reach on the top sections of their head.

2 Clear trolleys or equipment out of the way so that you get good all-round access (360°) to the client.

3 Keep your equipment close by so that you can reach them safely without putting you or the client at risk, and the items should be clean, sterile and ready for use.

Keeping work areas clean and safe to use at all times

Working efficiently, safely and effectively

Working efficiently and maximising your time is essential, so making the most of the resources available should occur naturally. One way of making the most of the shop's resources is being careful of how you handle the equipment and the products that you use. Always try to minimise waste, being careful of how much product you use.

Make full use of your time. Don't leave things to the last minute, because this will encroach on the barber's appointment time for the shave. Prepare the tools and

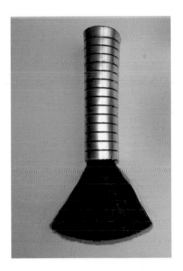

Even though you won't use the neck brush until the end of the service, make sure it's handy

EKU *statements*

GB1 (eku10) why it is important to position your tools, products and materials for ease of use

GB1 (eku13) why it is important to keep your work area clean and tidy

equipment so that they are cleaned and sterilised. Cleanliness is of paramount importance. The work area should be clean and free from clutter and waste items. Any used materials should be disposed of and not left out on the side. To do otherwise is:

- unprofessional, and shows that you are disorganised
- a hazard, as it presents a health risk to others – see the section on preventing infection, page 150.

You need to work in an orderly environment, with the materials and the equipment in position and ready for action. You need to be thinking about all of the things that you need **before** you need them. This is a good exercise in self-organisation and shows others that you are a true professional.

Activity

Answer the following questions in your portfolio. What is your shop's policy in respect to:

1 The safe disposal of sharp items?

2 The cleaning and maintenance of shaving materials?

3 Working safely within the shop?

4 Preparing the client prior to shaving?

Maintaining personal hygiene standards

Your personal hygiene

Personal hygiene is vitally important for anyone working in personal services. Your personal hygiene, or lack of it, will be immediately noticeable to everyone you come into contact with. You may have overslept, but if you haven't showered it will be very uncomfortable for you, your colleagues and the clients as **body odour** (BO) is unpleasant in any situation. Other strong smells are offensive too; the smells of nicotine or smoking are very off-putting to the client, particularly if they are a non-smoker. For more information on looking after your personal hygiene and general wellbeing, see Chapter 1, Make sure your own actions reduce risks to health and safety, page 120.

Cleaning tools and equipment

Tool preparation and maintenance

The tools that you use must always be sterilised and ready for use; the materials need to be kept close at hand, but well out of the way of clients and children. Any used disposable blades should be disposed of properly in the **sharps box**.

Brushes   Quality shaving brushes are made of pure badger bristle. The hair for the finest quality brush is taken from the neck of the animal and the natural texture and shape of the individual hairs provide a bristle that is coarse and stiff at the root end, whilst tapering slowly towards a soft, fine tip. The hairs from other areas of the animal are

---

EKU statements

GB1 (eku4) your own responsibilities under the current Control of Substances Hazardous to Health Regulations in relation to the use of shaving products

GB1 (eku15) the importance of personal hygiene

Remember

Bad breath is offensive to clients. Bad breath (**halitosis**) is the result of leaving particles to decay within the spaces between the teeth. Brush your teeth after every meal. Bad breath can also result from digestive troubles, stomach upsets, smoking and strong foods such as onion, garlic and some cheeses.

EKU statement

GB1 (eku16) methods of cleaning, disinfecting and/or sterilisation used in salons

Remember

Lathering brushes, sponges and bowls must be sterilised after each client.

used for lower quality brushes. Natural badger hair produces a brush that is both durable yet very flexible. There are 3 quality standards for badger brushes:

- **Pure** is a basic brush with short- to medium-length dark hair
- **Best** has medium- to long-length hairs and a creamy tip; it is slightly softer
- **Super** is a long-length bristle brush with a creamy tip and has better water retention properties than pure or best quality.

Other brushes are made of synthetic (man-made) materials such as nylon or acrylic.

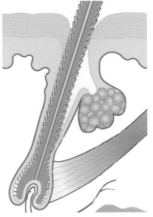

Cross-section of a hair follicle; drawing a sponge over the follicle will open it and allow for an easier shave

 Activity

Fill in the table below with the missing information.

Sterilising method	What tools and equipment is it used for?	How does it work?
Barbicide		
UV cabinet		
autoclave		

Bowls and mugs Traditionally, shaving bowls were made of polished chrome metal with a lid, or were made of wood. Modern versions are made of alloys or plastics that are lighter to hold and easier to clean and sterilise. Ceramic mugs are a popular alternative to bowls. Although they don't have the heat retention properties of metal bowls, they do have the benefit of having a handle and are therefore easier and possibly safer to hold when applying lather.

Sponges Sponges are used during sponge shaving. It is unlikely that you will be involved with assisting during the shave, but you will need to know how to prepare and clean them for the barber. Sponges are soaked in hot water and drawn over the face to open the beard follicles, just before the razor's blade sweeps over it; this allows coarser, heavier growth to be more easily removed.

Brush stands Shaving brush stands provide the ideal way of air drying lathering brushes. Wet brushes are placed on the stand so that the bristles point downwards. This will prevent the bristles from becoming misshapen, stop the bristles from developing mildew and rotting and prolong the life of the brush.

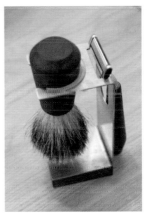

Never stand the brush on its end on the brush stand. If you do, the bristles will become misshapen and rot. Always point the bristles downwards!

Cleaning the equipment

Towels **Method of cleaning/sterilisation**: Large stocks of towels should be machine washed, dried and folded ready for use.

Shaving brush **Method of cleaning/sterilisation**: Wash in hot soapy water, flick dry and place on a brush stand to dry. Before they are used, they can be placed in the UV cabinet for 10 minutes.

Shaving bowls **Method of cleaning/sterilisation**: Wash in hot soapy water and dry. Then immerse in Barbicide™ or a bath of Cidex™ for 30 minutes. Alternatively, metal items can be sterilised in an autoclave for 20 minutes.

Shaving mugs **Method of cleaning/sterilisation**: Wash in hot soapy water and dry. Then immerse in Barbicide™ or a bath of Cidex™ for 30 minutes. Alternatively, sterilise in an autoclave for 20 minutes.

Remember

A wet, natural badger bristle brush should never be stood on its end and left to dry. The bristles will become misshapen and moisture will form mildew and rot. Always place a wet brush to air dry on a brush stand.

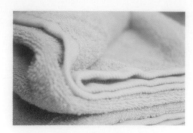

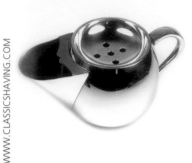

Brush stands and shaving brush holders Method of cleaning/sterilisation: Wash in hot soapy water and then dry. Metal stands can be placed in an autoclave for 20 minutes; plastic brush holders can be placed in a UV cabinet for 25 minutes.

Sponges Method of cleaning/sterilisation: Wash in hot soapy water and immerse in Barbicide™ jar for 30 minutes.

Avoiding cross-infestation and cross-infection

Infection and disease occurs by 2 obvious methods within the barber's shop environment. They can be either brought in by a "carrier" visiting the salon who then cross-infects other people within the salon or the result of poor hygiene and cleanliness within the salon. Most of the preparatory aspects covered in this chapter aim to keep the standards of hygiene within your working environment very high.

A humid environment can offer a perfect home for disease-carrying bacteria. If they can find food in the form of dust and dirt, they may reproduce rapidly. Good ventilation, however, provides a circulating air current that will help to prevent their growth. This is why it is important to keep the shop clean, dry and well aired at all times. This includes clothing, work areas, tools and all equipment.

Sterilisation provides the most effective way of providing hygienically safe work implements in salons; sterilisation destroys all living organisms. Different types of equipment use different sterilisation methods, which may be based on the use of heat, radiation or chemicals.

Ultraviolet radiation Ultraviolet (UV) radiation provides an alternative sterilising option. The items for sterilisation are placed in wall- or worktop-mounted cabinets fitted with UV-emitting light bulbs and exposed to the radiation for at least 15 minutes. If your scissors or combs are sterilised in a UV cabinet, remember to turn them over to make sure both sides have been done.

Chemical sterilisation Chemical sterilisers such as Barbicide™ or Cidex™ should be handled only with suitable personal protective equipment (PPE), as many of the solutions used are hazardous to health and should not come into contact with the skin. The most effective form of sterilisation is achieved by the total immersion of the contaminated implements into a jar or bath of these fluids.

Autoclave The autoclave provides a very efficient way of sterilising using heat. It is particularly good for metal tools, although the high temperatures are not suitable for plastic items such as brushes and combs. Items placed in the autoclave take around 20 minutes to sterilise – check with manufacturers' instructions for variations.

Activity
Copy the table below into your portfolio and then complete the activity by filling in the missing information.

Tools and equipment	How are they cleaned and maintained?
towels	
shaving bowls	
shaving brushes	
brush stands	
sponges	

Dealing with waste and shortages

Safe disposal of waste

There will always be some waste materials at the end of a shave. "Sharps" must be disposed of in a **sharps box**. Unused lather should be washed down the sink. It cannot be used again on another client because this may cause cross-infection. Towels need to be laundered and should be removed from the work area or placed into a covered towel bin prior to washing.

> **Remember**
>
> **Disposal of sharp items**
> Used razor blades and similar items should be placed into a safe container (**sharps box**), which must be clearly labelled and the top always re-tightened after disposal. When the container is full, it can be discarded. This type of salon waste should be kept away from general salon waste as special disposal arrangements may be provided by your local authority.

Low levels of materials

Look out for low levels of materials.

Towels   A busy barber's shop will go through a lot of towels during the day. When towels bins are full, or when clean stocks are starting to run low, make sure that more towels are put in the washing machine on the appropriate wash cycle. After washing, the towels must be dried and stored ready for use.

Neck strips   Neck strips are tucked in around the collar of gowns or cutting squares to stop bristle fragments falling into the client's clothes. Keep an eye on the neck strip dispenser and replace the roll when it is running low.

> **Remember**
>
> Barbers use a wide range of products that can be used in the shaving process. Keep an eye on the levels of stock and if you think that items are running low and you can't find them in stock, tell the person responsible for products so that new stock can be re-ordered.

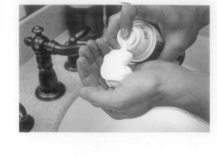

Learning about shaving products

Shaving oil

Shaving oils contain natural plant oils that moisturise the face whilst providing the perfect base for a close, comfortable shave. They are particularly suited to those with sensitive skins.

Application: Put 3–4 drops in the palm of your hand and then gently '"slap"' both palms together for 1–2 seconds before massaging the oil into the face. Let the oil '"work"' for at least 1 minute before applying the lather. Use this minute to wash the oil from your hands.

Shaving cream

Shaving creams moisturise the skin whilst providing good lubrication for the shave. Moisturising shaving creams can be used for all skin types, but normal to drier skins will benefit most from the creams.

Application: The cream is applied prior to the shave. Apply the cream thinly with fingertips to the area to be shaved, or lather up with a damp shaving brush and apply to the beard.

Shaving soap

Shaving soap provides the basic lubrication for a good close shave. Moisturising shaving soaps will create a rich, lubricating lather that softens and moisturises the skin.

Application: The soap is applied prior to the shave. Apply the cream thinly with fingertips to the area to be shaved, or lather up with a damp shaving brush and apply to the beard.

After shave balm

Shaving balms provide a moisturising effect that soothes and calms the skin after shaving. Moisturising balms are more suited for dry or sensitive skin types.

Application: Use a dab of the balm and massage gently onto the skin to assist absorption.

After shave lotion

Moisturising lotions replace lost oils and protect, cool and condition the skin after shaving. They are suitable for normal to dry skin types.

Application: Use a dab of the lotion and massage gently or pat onto the skin to assist absorption.

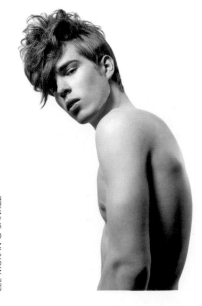

EKU *statement*

GB1 (eku12) the safety considerations which must be taken into account when using lathering products and hot towels

GB1 (eku17) the effect of hot and cold towels on the skin and hair

GB1 (eku18) the importance of lathering and its effect on skin and hair

Activity

Complete this activity by filling in the missing information.

Product	When is it applied?	How is it applied?
shaving oil		
shaving cream		
shaving soap		
after shave balm		
after shave lotion		

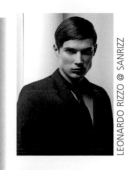

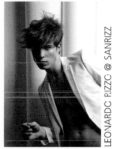

LEONARDO RIZZO @ SANRIZZ

LEONARDO RIZZO @ SANRIZZ

GB1.2 Prepare facial hair and skin for shaving services

The client's skin is prepared for shaving by cleansing and exfoliation, applying hot towels and applying the lather.

Cleansing and exfoliating the skin

The client's skin can be cleansed by washing with a mild soap or with a granular exfoliating face wash and water. Exfoliation is a process that will help remove the layer of dead cells that cover the face and lift the hairs into an upright position.

EKU *statement*

GB1 (eku20) how to prepare and use hot and cold towels

Remember

 An exfoliating face wash will deep clean and prepare the skin for shaving services.

Applying hot and cold towels

Prepare the skin and beard by applying hot towels to the face to ensure that the lather is applied to a warm face. Hot towels can be prepared by pre-heating in a warming cabinet or soaking them in a basin of hot water. After wringing out the excess water, they are placed around the facial area, but not covering the nose, to:

- soften the bristly hair
- cleanse the face
- open up the follicles
- prepare the skin for lathering.

Always make sure that the towels are not dripping wet and they are not too hot for the client. Check the temperature before applying the towels so that they are hot enough to prepare the skin but not too hot that they burn the client's skin.

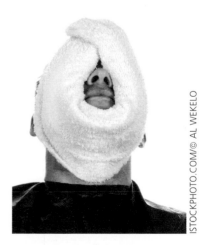

ISTOCKPHOTO.COM/© AL WEKELO

Avoid the client's nose when covering the client's face with a hot towel

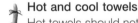

Activity

Different shops have different ways of doing things. Find out what your barber's shop procedures for maintaining towels are. Write down your answers in your portfolio.

1   At what point(s) in the day are towels washed?

2   What washing materials are used to wash the towels?

3   What wash cycle does the shop recommend?

4   How are the towels dried?

5   How are the towels stored and kept ready for use?

Remember

Hot and cool towels

Hot towels should not be used on a client with sensitive skin because this will irritate the skin further and prevent you from carrying out the service. Cool towels are used to soothe the face after shaving and to close the pores to finish the service. Cool towels should not be used on a client who is going to have a facial massage because this will close the pores prematurely and prevent the client from gaining the full benefit of the massage service.

EKU *statement*

GB1 (eku25) when, why and how to use brush and massage techniques when applying lathering products

Applying lathering products

Lathering

Remember

If you are applying lather by hand, wear close-fitting vinyl gloves. These will be more comfortable for the client and will stop your fingers slipping on the client's skin.

Traditionally lather was made up from soap and applied with a brush. Now they are formulated in a range of products that can be applied by brush or finger massage.

Lather is generally applied using a brush and bowl. It needs to be done quickly. Take particular care not to go beyond the extent of the beard as the barber will not be able to see the beard line beneath the lather. Do not cover the mouth, nose or go anywhere near the client's eyes. Alternatively, the lather can be applied by hand. Again, this needs to be done quickly and care must be taken during the application. The movements of the fingers use two massage techniques that are common to other hairdressing and barbering services: **effleurage** and **petrissage**.

EKU *statement*

GB1 (eku19) the function of effleurage and petrissage massage techniques when lathering

Massage techniques used in lathering   **Effleurage** is a light stroking movement applied with either the fingers or the palms of the hands. It is applied with an even, rhythmical movement with very little pressure to help create a feeling of relaxation. **Petrissage** is a pressing movement that lifts and compresses underlying structures of the skin. The pressure applied should be light, but firm enough to build up the richness of the lather and lift the bristles away from the skin.

Applying the lather

Preparing to lather

1 **Positioning** Adjusting the chair – recline the barber's chair and adjust the working height (and headrest) so that when you move around the chair, you can reach over the client's face without leaning or resting on them.

2 **Hygiene** Make sure that your hands are scrupulously clean. Place a clean tissue over the headrest to prevent the spread of infection from one head to another.

3 **Protection** Put a clean, fresh gown or cutting square on the client.

4 **Cleansing** Cleanse the client's skin in preparation for the massage service. Exfoliate if needed

5 **Hot towels** Apply a hot towel to the client's face to open up the pores in preparation for the massage. Remove the towel before it goes cold.

Lathering A rich lather is achieved by using a shaving brush or your fingers and should be applied quickly.

- Build up a rich lather with the brush and apply in small circular motions all over the skin, but not extending beyond the area of beard hair. The movements should lift the beard; go in a direction against the lie of the hair to produce the best results.

- Apply the lather to one area of the beard at a time, not all over the beard area of the face; this prevents the skin from drying out.

- Take up to 3 or 4 minutes to apply and build up the lather; this will produce the best results for the shave.

- Inform the barber that the client is ready.

Telling the barber when the client is prepared

Prepare for the shave so that it fits in with the barber's other tasks and duties. There is no point starting any part of the process too soon because the benefits of what you are doing will be lost. Hot towels start cooling from the point that they are applied. If too much heat is lost prior to lathering, the follicles will start to close and the effectiveness of the shave will be lost. Similarly, the lather should be applied to a warm face to lubricate the surface of the skin and lift the facial hair. All of these are critical for the quality of the shave. Always make sure that you work with the barber and only start the preparation process when you have been told to. The moment the client is ready for shaving, let the barber know.

Removing lather and cooling the skin

The final stage of the shaving process is to cool the skin and close the hair follicles. Before this can happen, any remaining lather must be removed using a damp towel or sponge. "Pat" the face dry, taking care not to drag or pull the skin because the client's skin can still be quite sensitive.

Now apply a cool towel, which can be prepared by pre-soaking in basin of cold water. Take the towel out of the basin and wring out the excess moisture. Apply in a similar way

Remember

 Pre-soak towels in a basin of hot water; then wring out the excess water and place around the face (do not cover the nose). Hot towels open up the follicles and prepare the skin for massage. Ensure that the towels are not dripping wet and they are not too hot.

EKU *statement*

GB1 (eku23) why timing is critical to the shaving service

EKU *statement*

GB1 (eku26) how to remove lathering products effectively and why this is important

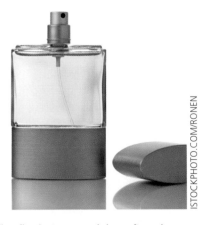

The final step: applying after shave

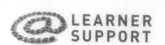

to hot towels, so that the nose is not covered. Leave for a few minutes and then remove the towels and place them in the towel bin.

Finally, complete the service by applying a little talcum powder (this dries the skin and prevents chapping), and the application of either an after shave balm or lotion. An after shave balm is more suitable to drier skin types because it helps to moisturise and lubricate the skin. A lotion can also be used; this is more "zesty" and suitable for normal to oily skin types.

Remember

Ask the client how cold they would like the cool towel to be. It can be a shock if the towel is very cold on an already warmed face.

EKU *statement*

GB1 (eku24) the types and causes of problems that may occur when assisting with shaving services

Problems that you may encounter

Problem	Possible cause
client's skin is burned	● hot towels were not wrung out properly before application ● hot towels too hot
client develops rash after the shave	● tools not cleaned and sterilised properly ● sterilising chemicals not rinsed off equipment properly ● client has in-growing hairs from shaving curly hair too closely ● wrong shaving products applied ● shaving products applied wrongly
uneven, patchy shave result	● hot towels not applied ● hot towels allowed to cool down too much before shave is carried out ● poor or uneven lather application
client's skin sensitive after shave	● skin not allowed to cool properly ● cool towels were not applied ● shave was too close ● poor or uneven lather application ● talcum not applied ● wrong shaving products applied ● shaving products applied wrongly

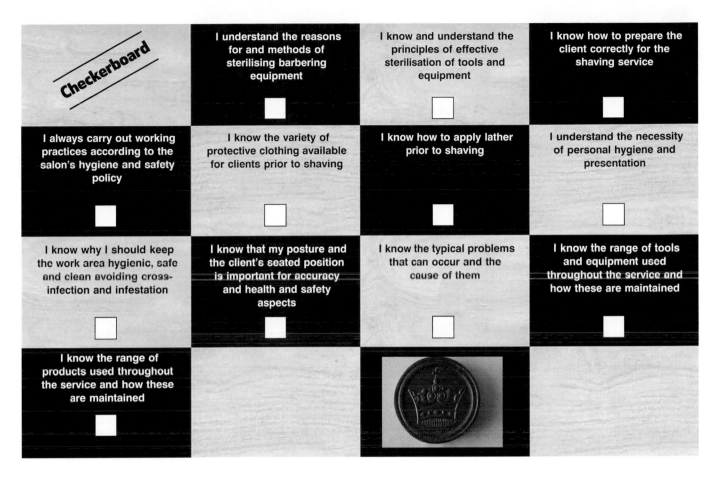

Checkerboard

I understand the reasons for and methods of sterilising barbering equipment ☐	**I know and understand the principles of effective sterilisation of tools and equipment** ☐	**I know how to prepare the client correctly for the shaving service** ☐
I always carry out working practices according to the salon's hygiene and safety policy ☐	**I know the variety of protective clothing available for clients prior to shaving** ☐	**I know how to apply lather prior to shaving** ☐	**I understand the necessity of personal hygiene and presentation** ☐
I know why I should keep the work area hygienic, safe and clean avoiding cross-infection and infestation ☐	**I know that my posture and the client's seated position is important for accuracy and health and safety aspects** ☐	**I know the typical problems that can occur and the cause of them** ☐	**I know the range of tools and equipment used throughout the service and how these are maintained** ☐
I know the range of products used throughout the service and how these are maintained ☐			

Revision questions

Q1 Fill in the blank: The _____ massage technique is described as a light stroking movement applied with either the fingers or the palms of the hands.

Q2 Exfoliation removes the build up of dead skin cells. True or false?

Q3 Which of the following are features of after shave balms? (You may choose more than one answer.)

1 cool the skin
2 exfoliate the skin
3 moisturise the skin
4 prepare the skin for shaving
5 soothe the skin after shaving
6 should be applied with hot towels

Q4 A "badger" brush is made of real badger hair. True or false?

Q5 Which is the finest quality "real hair" shaving brush? (Choose one answer.)

a pure bristle
b best quality
c super quality
d nylon bristle

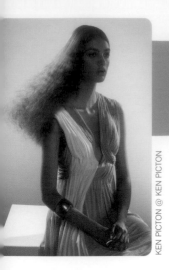

Appendix 1 Health and safety legislation

This section will provide you with an outline of the main health and safety regulations that affect hairdressers and barbers in their work.

Management of Health and Safety at Work Regulations 1999

The main regulation requires the employer to appoint competent personnel to conduct risk assessments for the health and safety of all staff working on the premises as well as other visitors to the business premises. Staff must be adequately trained to take appropriate action, and eliminate or minimise any risks. Other regulations cover the necessity of setting up procedures for emergency situations and reviewing the risk assessment processes. In salons where 5 or more people are employed, there is the added obligation to set up a system for monitoring health surveillance, should the risk assessments identify a need.

The main requirements for management of health and safety are:

- identify any potential hazards
- assess the risks which could arise from these hazards identifying who is at risk
- eliminate or minimise the risks
- train staff to identify and control risks
- regularly review the assessment processes.

Young workers at risk

There is also a requirement to carry out a risk assessment for young people. Any staff member who is under school-leaving age must have a personalised risk assessment kept on file. This is also applicable for those on work experience or Saturday staff.

- easy online steps to control health risks from chemicals
- COSHH Essentials has been developed to help firms comply with the COSHH regulations. The COSHH Essentials Website is easy to use and is available free as part of **hsedirect** – a database of all health and safety legislation and HSE's priced guidance. Available at http://www.coshhessentials.org.uk/.

Workplace (Health, Safety and Welfare) Regulations 1992

These regulations supersede the Offices, Shops and Railway Premises Act 1963 (OSRPA) and cover the following workplace key points:

- maintenance of the workplace and the equipment in it
- ventilation, temperature and lighting
- cleanliness

- sanitary and washing facilities
- drinking water supply
- resting, eating and changing facilities
- storage of clothing
- glazing
- traffic routes
- work space.

Amendments and additions in this regulation provide new requirements for employers with particular attention for glazed areas such as windows and doors, etc. Any transparent and translucent partitions must be made of safe materials and if they could cause injury to anyone, they should be appropriately marked. Other amendments have particular rules for rest rooms and rest areas. These must include suitable alternative arrangements to protect non-smokers from the effects caused by tobacco smoke and suitable rest facilities for any person at work who is either pregnant or a nursing mother.

Health and Safety (First-Aid) Regulations 1981

The Health and Safety (First-Aid) Regulations 1981 require the employer to provide adequate and appropriate equipment, facilities and personnel to enable first aid to be given to their employees if they are injured or become ill at work.

The minimum first-aid provision on any work site is:

- a suitably stocked first-aid box
- an appointed person to take charge of first-aid arrangements.

It is also important to remember that accidents can happen at any time. First-aid provision needs to be available at all times people are at work.

Personal Protective Equipment (PPE) at Work Regulations 1992

These relate to the requirement of employers to provide suitable and sufficient protective clothing and equipment for all employees to use. The PPE Regulations 1992 require managers to make an assessment of the processes and activities carried out at work and to identify where and when special items of clothing should be worn. In hairdressing environments, the potential hazards and dangers revolve around the task of providing hairdressing services – that is, in general, the application of hairdressing treatments and associated products.

Potentially hazardous substances used by hairdressers include:

- acidic solutions of varying strengths
- caustic alkaline solutions of varying strengths
- flammable liquids, which are often in pressurised containers
- vapours
- dyeing compounds.

There are also potentially hazardous items of equipment and their individual applications, such as:

- electrical appliances
- heated/heating instruments
- sharp cutting tools.

All these items require correct handling and safe usage procedures, and for several of them this includes the wearing of suitable items of protective equipment. Remember that not wearing appropriate gloves can lead to dermatitis (see page 25).

Control of Substances Hazardous to Health (COSHH) Regulations 2003

Hairdressing employers are required by law to make an assessment of the exposure to all the substances used in their salon that could be potentially hazardous to themselves, their employees and other salon visitors, who may be affected by the work activity. The purpose of COSHH regulations is to make sure that people are working in the safest possible environment and conditions.

A substance is considered to be hazardous if it can cause harm to the body. It only presents a risk if it is:

- in contact with the skin or eyes
- absorbed through the skin or via the eyes (either directly or from contact from with contaminated surfaces or clothing)
- inhaled (breathed in from the atmosphere)
- ingested via contaminated food or fingers
- injected
- introduced to the body via cuts and abrasions.

Cosmetic Products (Safety) Regulations 2008

These regulations lay down the recommended volumes and percentage strengths of different hydrogen-based products. The strength will vary depending on whether it has been produced for professional or non-professional use. It is important that the manufacturer's guidance material and current legislation is checked when using or selling products.

Health and Safety (Information for Employees) Regulations 1989

This regulation requires the employer to make available to all employees, notices, posters and leaflets either in the approved format or those actually published by the HSE.

Health and Safety (Display Screen Equipment) Regulations 1992

These regulations cover the use of computers and similar equipment in the workplace. Although not generally high risk, prolonged use can lead to eye strain, mental stress and possible muscular pain. As more hairdressing salons use information technology and computers this is becoming a major consideration for hairdressing employees.

It is the employer's duty to assess display screen equipment and reduce the risks that are discovered. They will need to plan the scheduling of work so that there are regular breaks or changes in activity and provide information training for the equipment users. Computer users will also be entitled to eyesight tests, which will be paid for by the employer.

Manual Handling Operations Regulations 1992

These regulations apply in all occupations where manual lifting occurs. They require employers to carry out a risk assessment of the work processes and activities that involve lifting. The risk assessment should address detailed aspects of the following:

- any risk of injury
- the manual movement that is involved in the task
- the physical constraints the loads incur
- the work environmental constraints that are incurred
- the worker's individual capabilities
- steps and/or remedial action to take in order to minimise the risk.

Provision and Use of Work Equipment Regulations (PUWER) 1998

These regulations refer to the regular maintenance and monitoring of work equipment. Any equipment, new or second-hand, must be suitable for the purpose that it is intended. In addition to this, they require that anyone using this equipment must be adequately trained.

Electricity at Work Regulations 1989

These regulations require employers to maintain electrical equipment in a safe condition and to have it checked by a suitably qualified person. A written record of testing must be kept and made available for inspection. It is the employees' responsibility for reporting any known faulty equipment to their employer or supervisor. The following information must be kept:

- the electrician's/contractor's name, address, contact details
- an itemised list of salon electrical equipment along with serial number (for individual identification)
- the date of inspection
- the date of purchase/disposal.

Reporting of Injuries, Diseases and Dangerous Occurrences Regulations 1995 (RIDDOR)

Under these regulations there are certain diseases and groups of infections that, if sustained at work, are noticeable by law. So if any employees suffer a personal injury at work which results in one of the following, they must be reported to the appropriate authority:

- death
- major injuries, including: fractures (not fingers and toes) amputation, dislocation, loss of sight and other eye injuries
- more than 24 hours in hospital
- an incapacity to work for more than 3 calendar days.

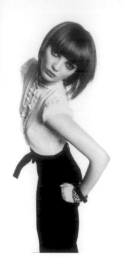

Appendix 2 People's rights and consumer legislation

Equal opportunities

The Equal Opportunities Commission (EOC) has the statutory duty to:

- work towards the elimination of discrimination
- promote equality of opportunity between men and women (and in relation to persons undergoing gender reassignment)
- keep the relevant legislation under review.

The legislation within the remit of the EOC is wide ranging; however, the main considerations are:

- equal pay
- sex discrimination
- disability discrimination (summary below).

In general, the **Sex Discrimination Act** (SDA) requires goods, facilities and services, whether for payment or not, which are offered to the public, to be provided on the same basis for both sexes. The SDA prohibits direct and indirect sex discrimination.

Direct sex discrimination is treating a woman less favourably than a man (or vice versa) because of their gender.

Indirect sex discrimination occurs when a condition or requirement is applied equally to both women and men but, in fact, it affects more women than men (or vice versa) and is not justifiable on objective grounds unrelated to sex. The Act provides for exceptions, but unless a relevant exception to the requirements of the SDA can be used, facilities and services should be open to both sexes in the same way.

For more information, visit www.eoc.org.uk/index.asp.

Disability Discrimination Act 2005 (DDA 2005)

This Act makes it unlawful to discriminate against disabled persons in connection with employment, the provision of goods, facilities and services or the disposal or management of premises; makes provision about the employment of disabled persons; and establishes a National Disability Council.

The Act protects the rights of disabled people and new revisions in 2005 have particular relevance to the business proprietor. For more information on this or other accessibility issues, visit www.disability.gov.uk/legislation.

Data Protection Act 1998

Your clients have the following rights, which can be enforced through any county court:

- **Right of subject access** – This is the right to find out what information about them is held on computer and in some paper records.

- **Correcting inaccurate data** – They have the right to have inaccurate personal data rectified, blocked, erased or destroyed. If your client believes that they have suffered damage or distress as a result of the processing of inaccurate data they can ask the court to award compensation.

- **Preventing junk mail** (from salons that market to their customer base) – Your client has the right to request in writing that a data controller does not use your personal data for direct marketing by post (sometimes known as "junk mail"), by telephone or by fax.

For more information on consumer rights in relation to the Data Protection Act, visit www. informationcommissioner.gov.uk/.

Remember

Data Protection Act 1998
The Data Protection Act (DPA) applies to any business that uses computers or paper-based systems for storing personal information about its clients and staff.

It places obligations on the person holding the information (data controller) to deal with it properly.

It gives the person that the information concerns (data subject) rights regarding the data held about them.

The duties of the data controller
There are eight principles put in place by the DPA to make sure that data is handled correctly. By law, the data controller must keep to these principles. The principles say that the data must be:

- fairly and lawfully processed

- processed for limited purposes

- adequate, relevant and not excessive

- accurate

- not kept for longer than is necessary

- processed in line with your rights

- secure

- not transferred to other countries without adequate protection.

For more information, see http://www.ico.gov.uk/.

Sale of Goods Act 1979 and Sale and Supply of Goods Act 1994

The Sale of Goods Act 1979 and the later Sale and Supply of Goods Act 1994 are the main legal instruments helping buyers to obtain redress when their purchases go wrong. It is in the interest of anyone who sells goods or services to understand the implications of these Acts and the responsibilities they have under them. Essentially, these Acts state that what you sell must fit its description, be fit for its purpose and be of satisfactory quality. If not, you – as the supplier – are obliged to sort out the problem.

Briefly, these Acts requires the vendor:

- To make sure that goods **conform to contract**. This means that they must be as you describe them, e.g. highlight shampoo stops your highlights from fading.
- The goods must also be of **satisfactory quality**, meaning they should be safe, work properly and have no defects.
- You must also ensure the goods are **fit for purpose**. This means they should be capable of doing what they're meant for. For example, in the case of a brush it shouldn't fall apart when it is first used.

Consumer Protection Act 1987

This Act follows European laws to protect the buyer in the following areas:

- product liability – a customer may claim compensation for a product that doesn't reach general standards of safety
- general safety requirements – it is a criminal offence to sell goods that are unsafe; traders that breach this conduct may face fines or even imprisonment
- misleading prices – misleading consumers with wrongly displayed prices is also an offence.

The Act is designed to help safeguard the consumer from products that do not reach reasonable levels of safety. Your salon will take adequate precautions in procuring, using and supplying reputable products and maintaining them so that they remain in good condition.

Prices Act 1974

The price of products has to be displayed in order to prevent a false impression to the buyer.

Trades Descriptions Act 1968 and 1972

Products must not be falsely or misleadingly described in relation to their quality, fitness, price or purpose, by advertisements, orally, in displays or in descriptions. And, since 1972, it has also been a requirement to label a product clearly, so that the buyer can see where the product was made.

Briefly, a retailer cannot:

- mislead consumers by making false statements about products
- offer sale products at half price unless they have been offered at the actual price for a reasonable length of time.

Resale Prices Act 1964 and 1976

Manufacturers can supply a recommended price (MRRP or manufacturers' recommended retail price), but the seller is not obliged to sell at the recommended price.

Answers to revision questions

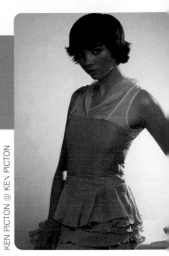

KEN PICTON @ KEN PICTON

Chapter**one**

Q1	harm
Q2	True
Q3	1 3 6
Q4	True
Q5	D

Chapter**two**

Q1	clients
Q2	True
Q3	1 2 5 6
Q4	True
Q5	4

Chapter**three**

Q1	confidential
Q2	True
Q3	4 6
Q4	True
Q5	B

Chapter**four**

Q1	infestation
Q2	True
Q3	4 5
Q4	False
Q5	C

Chapter**five**

Q1	removing
Q2	False
Q3	1 4
Q4	False
Q5	C

Chapter**six**

Q1	sterilised
Q2	True
Q3	1 5
Q4	True
Q5	B

Chapter**seven**

Q1	fade
Q2	True
Q3	2 3
Q4	True
Q5	A

Chapter**eight**

Q1	fix
Q2	True
Q3	1 2 3
Q4	True
Q5	C

Chapter**nine**

Q1	Traction
Q2	True
Q3	1 3
Q4	True
Q5	C

Chapter**ten**

Q1	dissolve
Q2	False
Q3	2 3 4 5
Q4	True
Q5	B

Chapter**eleven**

Q1	effleurage
Q2	True
Q3	1 3 5
Q4	True
Q5	C

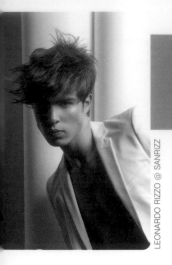

Useful addresses and websites

Business

Arbitration, Conciliation and Advisory Service (ACAS)

Head Office, Brandon House,
180 Borough High Street, London, SE1 1LW

T: 020 7210 3613

www.acas.org.uk

Helpline 08457 47 47 47

Hairdressing Employers' Association (HEA)

10 Coldbath Square, London, EC1R 5HL

T: 020 7833 0633

Training & Education

Hairdressing and Beauty Industry Authority (Habia)

Oxford House, Sixth Avenue, Sky Business Park,
Robin Hood Airport, Doncaster, DN9 3GG

T: 08452 306080

www.habia.org

Association of Hairdressing Teachers (AHT)

5 Viscount Gardens, Byfleet, Surrey, KT14 6HE

City & Guilds (C&G)

1 Giltspur Street, London, EC1A 9DD

T: 020 7294 2800

www.city-and-guilds.co.uk

Department for Education and Skills

www.dfes.gov.uk

Lifelong Learning

www.lifelonglearning.co.uk

Qualifications and Curriculum Authority (QCA)

83 Piccadilly, London, W1J 8QA

T: 020 7509 3097

www.qca.org.uk

The Institute of Trichologists

Ground Floor office, 24 Langroyd Road,
London, SW17 7PL

T: 08706 070602

www.trichologists.org.uk

Vocational Training Charitable Trust (VTCT)

3rd Floor. Eastleigh House.
Upper Market Street. Eastleigh

www.vtct.org.uk

World Federation of Hairdressing and Beauty Schools

PO Box 367, Coulsdon, Surrey, CR5 2TP

T: 01737 551355

World Federation of Hairdressing Schools

73 Marlpit Lane, Coulsdon, Surrey, CR5 2HF

Publication

Hairdressers Journal International (HJ)

Quadrant House, The Quadrant, Sutton,
Surrey, SM2 5AS

T: 020 8652 3500

www.reedbusiness.com

Creative Head

Mallan House, Bridge End, Hexham,
Northumberland, NE46 4DQ

www.head1st.net

Black Beauty and Hair

Culvert House, Culvert Road, London, SW11

T: 020 7720 2108

www.blackbeauty.co.uk

Trade associations

British Association of Beauty Therapy and Cosmetology Limited (BABTAC)

Meteor Court, Barnett Way, Barnwood, Gloucester, GL4 3GG

Caribbean and Afro Society of Hairdressers (CASH)

42 North Cross Road, East Dulwich, London, SE22 8PY

T: 020 8299 2859

Commission for Racial Equality

Elliot House, 10–12 Allington Street, London, SW1E 5EH

T: 020 7828 7022

www.cre.gov.uk

Cosmetic, Toiletry and Perfumery Association (CTPA)

Josaron House, 5–7 John Princes Street, London, W1G 0JN

T: 020 7491 8891

www.ctpa.org.uk

Fellowship for British Hairdressing

Bloxham Mill, Barford Road, Bloxham, Banbury, Oxon

T: 01295 724579

Freelance Hair and Beauty Federation

6 Warleigh Road, Brighton, East Sussex, BN1 4TN

T: 01273 604556

www.fhbf.org.uk

Guild of Hairdressers (GUILD)

Unit 1E, Redbrook Business Park, Wilthorpe Road, Barnsley, S75 1JN

T: 01226 730112

Hairdressing and Beauty Suppliers' Association (HBSA)

Bedford Chambers, The Piazza, Covent Garden, London, WC2E 8HA

T: 020 7836 4008

Hairdressing and Beauty Suppliers Association

1st Floor, Manfield House, 1 Southampton Street, Covent Garden, London, WC2R OLR

Hairdressing Council (HC)

12 David House, 45 High Street, South Norwood, London, SE25 6HJ

T: 020 8771 6205

www.haircouncil.org.uk

Health and Beauty Employers Federation (part of the Federation of Holistic Therapists)

18 Shakespeare Business Centre, Hathaway Close, Eastleigh, Hampshire, SO50 4SR

www.fht.org.uk

Incorporated Guild of Hairdressers, Wigmakers and Perfumers

Unit 8, Vulcan Road, M1, Distribution Centre, Meadowhall, Sheffield, S9 1EW

National Hairdressers' Federation (NHF)

One Abbey Court, Fraser Road, Priory Business Park, Bedford, MK44 3WH

www.the-nhf.org

Legal and regulatory

Health and Safety Executive

Publications
PO Box 1999, Sudbury, Suffolk, CO10 6FS
(HSE) Infoline

T: 0845 345 0055

www.hse.gov.uk

Equal Opportunities Commission

Arndale House, Arndale Centre, Manchester, M4 3EQ

T: 0161 833 9244

Union of Shop, Distributive and Allied Workers (USDAW)

188 Wilmslow Road, Fallowfield, Manchester, M14 6LJ

T: 0161 224 2804

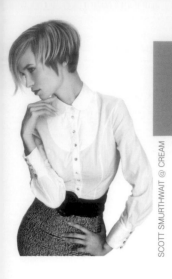

SCOTT SMURTHWAIT @ CREAM

Glossary

Accident book a record of accidents within the workplace required by health and safety law

Alpha keratin the state the hair is in before stretching and setting into a new shape

Ammonium thioglycolate an alkaline substance in perm lotions that reacts with the disulphide bonds

Anti-oxidant conditioner stops the oxidation process of chemical services

Antiseptics reduces the growth of micro-organisms that cause disease

Appointment system the efficient way of organising salon work

Appraisal A process of reviewing work performance over a period of time

Bacteria a tiny organism that can only be seen under a microscope

Barrier cream a cream that protects the skin against harmful moisture, or infection

Beta keratin the state the hair is in after it has been stretched and set into a new shape

Body language non-verbal communication provided by gestures, expressions and mannerisms

Body odour (BO) the result of poor personal hygiene and lack of regular washing

Cane rows see **Cornrows**

Client care maintaining goodwill whilst developing regular, repeated business

Cold-fusion hair extensions a system of connecting hair extensions by using adhesives and adhesive strips

Confidentiality the professional way of handling client information

Congo plait see **French plait**

Cornrows (also known as cane rows) a term used to describe an effect created by multiple rows of plaits that follow the contour of the head

Cortex the inner part of the hair where most chemical processes take place

COSHH an abbreviation for Control of Substances Hazardous to Health; these are health and safety regulations affecting you in your work

Cross-infection the transmission of infectious micro-organisms from one person to another

Cross-infestation the transmission of animal parasites from one person to another

Cuticle the outer protective layer of the hair resembling overlapping tiles on a roof

Dermatitis an occupational disease that affects the skin causing an itching sensation accompanied by reddening and dry cracked areas

Disinfection does not kill all organisms like sterilisation, but slows down the rate of growth of bacteria

Disulphide bonds the chemical bonds within the hair that are rearranged during perming and neutralising

Effective communication professional communication that is not ambiguous, providing clear instruction or information

Effleurage a light stroking movement applied with either the fingers or the palms of the hands

Emulsify a way of mixing the colour with water in order to remove it from the hair

Exfoliate to scrub skin with a gritty substance to remove the dead cells of the surface layer

French plait (also known as Congo plait/Guinea plait) a 3-strand plait that starts, centrally, near the front hairline and continues closely to the scalp to the nape and continues as a freely hanging plait beyond

Friction a firm, vigorous rubbing massage technique made by the fingertips, used during shampooing

Goodwill the reputation of a business formed by the people who work for it

Guinea plait see **French plait**

Hair trap a flexible nylon or plastic plug that helps to stop hair from entering the drain

Halitosis bad breath

Hazard something with potential to cause harm

Hot-bonded hair extensions a system of connecting hair extensions by using resin or hard plastics

Humidity the moisture level in the air

Hydrophilic water loving
Hydrophobic water repelling

Legislation laws created by parliament

Medulla the central part of the hair that is only found in coarser hair types
Melanin the naturally occurring pigments formed within the skin and hair
Moisturising balms cooling, soothing and moisture replenishing lotions applied after shaving to counteract the abrasive effects of the process

Neutraliser a chemical compound which is used to both balance and fix hair that has been previously permed
NVQ an abbreviation for National Vocational Qualification: job-ready qualifications at a range of different levels

Pathogen something that can cause disease, e.g. a bacterium or a virus
Personal development plan an ongoing action plan for self-improvement that defines personal objectives or targets, set over a period of time (often reviewed during appraisal)
Petrissage a kneading movement of the skin that lifts and compresses underlying structures of the skin, often used when applying conditioner
pH balance the natural acid mantle of skin and hair at pH5.5
pH level a measurement of a solution that denotes whether it is alkaline (pH 8–14), or acid (pH 6–1)
Pigment a granular form of colouration that can be natural or artificial
Practice block a modelling head with longer hair that can be attached to a work surface for practicing techniques

Removal solution a chemical formulated to dissolve the adhesive connecting the hair extension to the hair in cold-fusion systems
Removal tool a metal pair of pliers used for breaking the bond connecting the hair extension to the hair in hot-bonded systems
Revenue stream a source of income that comes into a business, e.g. retail sales, sales of services, sales of treatments
Risk assessment the process of assessing hazards within the workplace
Risk the likelihood of a hazard's potential being realised
Rotary a quicker and firmer circulatory movement used in shampooing.

Senegalese twists a twisting technique that resembles the plaited effect created by cornrows
Sharps the name given to sharp items, e.g. razor blades
Sharps box a designated sealed container used for the safe disposal of sharp items, e.g. used razor blades
Sterilisation the complete eradication of living organisms
Stock rotation when shelves are re-stocked the newer product is put at the back and the older stock is brought to the front; to be sold first
Surface conditioner a light conditioner that works on the outside of the hair to smooth and fill areas of damaged, missing or worn cuticle until next shampoo

Traction alopecia a condition that is caused by the excessive pulling of hair at the root, it is often associated with longer hair worn in plaits, twists, hair ups and extensions

Virgin hair a hairdressing term describing hair that has not been coloured

Index

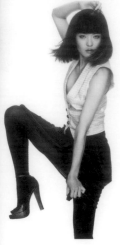

absorption 68
accelerators 60
accident book 5, 18
accidents 18
  see also emergencies
additions 133
  see also extensions
aloe vera shampoo 71
alpha keratin 81, 87
ammonium thioglycolate 107, 108
angry clients 48
anti-oxidant conditioner 66, 77, 104
appeal/grievance procedure 34–5
appointment system 37, 45
appointments 45–8
  drop in 46
  offer alternatives 43
  recording information 46–8
  service timings 47
  telephone calls 46
appraisal 24, 32–4
assembly points 16
attraction 68
autoclave 15

backwash 61
bacteria 56
bad breath (halitosis) 5, 20
barrier cream 20, 53
basin 61
behaviour 21
beta keratin 81, 87
blockages 61
blow dryers 85–6
blow drying 81–95
  apply styling/finishing
    products 88–9
  checklist 86
  dos and don'ts 95
  finger drying 94
  focusing jet stream 91
  following instructions 87
  how it works 87
  long hair step-by-step 93–4
  position client/self 82

roots to points 91
short hair step-by-step 92–3
tensioned hair 92
timing 86
tools/equipment 82–5
body language 24, 25
body odour (BO) 5, 20
breakages 14
brushes 83–5
  bristles 84
  Denman 84
  handles 84
  paddle 85
  round 85
  shaving 148–9
  vented 84–5

camomile shampoo 71
cane rows 126
cap highlights 99
  removing 101
chairs 63
chemical sterilisation 15
chemicals
  handling 12
clarifying shampoo 71
clay 89
cleaning
  accelerators 60
  basin/backwash area 61, 69
  floors 63
  hood dryers 60
  mirrors 59
  seating 63
  shaving tools and equipment 149–50
  steamers 60–1
  styling tools 60
  work surfaces 63
client
  confidentiality 44, 57
  difficult/angry 48
  gowning 13
  hanging coats/jackets 27
  needs 26
  personal belongings 26–7
  positioning 68–9
  protective equipment 13
client care 37, 40–2
  communication 25–6
  confidentiality 44, 57

difficult/angry clients 48
first impressions 27–8, 38
good 40–2
providing help 27
client records 57–8
clothes 19
coconut shampoo 71
cold-fusion extensions 133
  removal 140–1
colour
  full head 99
  lightener 98
  permanent 98
  quasi-permanent 98
  removal 101–4
  semi-permanent 98
  T-section 99
  waste disposal 58–9, 100
colouring 97–105
  cap highlights 99, 101
  emulsifying 102–3
  faults/solutions 102
  materials 55
  meche/foil highlights 99
  multiple colour removal 103–4
  position client/self 99
  re-growth 99
  removing colour 101–4
  single colour removal 102
  slices 99
  techniques 98–9
communication
  body language 25
  good 25, 29
  listening 25
  posture and gestures 26
  tone of voice 42
condition of hair 87
conditioner
  absorption 68
  anti-oxidant 77, 103
  attraction 68
  benefits of 76
  how it works 67–8
  surface 66, 77
  treatment/penetrating 77
  types of 77
conditioning 66–7, 72, 76–8
  after a perm 113
  after colouring 104
  following instructions 72, 76

positioning client/self 68–9
products and equipment 72
rinsing/finishing 78
step by step 77
confidence 25
confidentiality 37, 44, 57
Consumer Protection Act (1987) 164
Control of Substances Hazardous to Health
(COSHH) Regulations (2003) 12,
59, 160
cornrows 118, 126–7
cortex 77, 81, 87
Cosmetic Products (Safety) Regulations
(1989) 160
cross-infection 14–15, 53
cross-infestation 14–15, 53
customer care see client care
cuticle 77, 81, 87

Data Protection Act (1998) 44, 57, 163
defining crème 88–9
Denman brush 84
dermatitis 5, 12, 20
detangling 82
detergent 67
difficult clients 48
diffuser 85
Disability Discrimination Act (DDA)
(2005) 162
disease 14–15
disinfection 53
disposal of sharps 11
disposal of waste 58–9
disulphide bonds 107, 108
double twists 118
dress code 27–8
see also personal appearance
dryers
hand 85–6
hood 60, 72

effective communication 37
see also communication
effleurage 66, 73, 154
electric shock 15
electrical appliances 15–16
Electricity at Work Regulations
(1989) 161
electricity, working safely with 15–16
emergencies 16
evacuation 16–17
fire 16–17
empathy 25
emulsifying 97, 102–3
emulsion 67
enquires 41–2
equal opportunities 162
Equal Opportunities Commission
(EOC) 162
eumelanin 98
exfoliate 145

extensions 132–43
additions 133
client comfort 139
cold-fusion removal 140–1
cold-fusion systems 133
enhancements 133
hot-bonded removal 142
hot-bonded systems 133
maintenance 134
plaited/braided 133
position client/self 135–6
real hair 138
removal 134–43
removal solutions 132, 138
removal tools 132, 138
risks 136
sewn-in 133
sewn-in removal 143
synthetic (artificial) hair 137–8

feet 20
finger drying 94
finishing products see styling/finishing
products
fire safety 16–17
causes of fire 16
evacuation rules 16–17
fire exits 16
fire extinguisher colour codes 17
fire fighting equipment 16–17
raising the alarm 16
types of fire 17
first aid box 18
fixing spray 123
floors 63
foils 99
removing 102
French plait 118, 125–6
friction 66, 73
full head colour 99
fungi 56

gel 89, 123
gestures 26
glaze 89, 123
goodwill 24
gowning 13
greeting clients 42, 46
grievance procedure 34–5
grips 55

hair
condition 87
structure 77
hair clippings
disposal of 58
hair extensions see extensions
hair trap 53, 61
hairspray 88, 90
halitosis (bad breath) 5, 20

handling chemicals 12
hands 20
hazard 5
hazard and risk 6–7
hazards 6–8, 13–14
environmental 6
equipment/materials 6
examples of 6
personal 7
head lice 15
health and hygiene
personal 20–1
health and safety 5–21
being responsible 7–8
concerns/questions 8
cross-infection/infestation 14–15
employer's/employee's duties 10
handling chemicals 12
hazard and risk 6–7
legislation 5, 158–64
manual handling 11–12
notices/procedures 9
personal protective equipment (PPE)
12–13
preventing infection 14–15
reducing risk 9–16
responsibilities 5
sharps disposal 11
slips and trips 13–14
spillage/breakages 14
sterilisation 15
waste disposal 11
work routines 7
working safely 11–18
working with electricity 15–16
Health and Safety at Work Act (HASAWA)
(1974) 10
Health and Safety (Display Screen
Equipment) Regulations
(1992) 160
Health and Safety Executive (HSE) 5
Health and Safety (First Aid) Regulations
(1981) 159
Health and Safety (Information for
Employees) Regulations (1989) 160
hood dryer 60, 72
hot-bonded extensions 133
removal 142
humidity 81, 87
hydrophilic 66, 67
hydrophobic 66, 67
hygiene
personal 20–1

infection
preventing 14–15
ionic attraction 68

jewellery 19
job description 33–4
jojoba shampoo 71

lathering 154–6
learning and development 31–5
   appraisal/review 32–4
   asking for feedback 31–2
   self-assessment 31
   targets 33–4
legislation 5, 158–64
lemon shampoo 71
lifting see manual handling
lightener 98
limits of authority 30
listening 25
long hair
   blow drying 93–4

maintenance
   hair extensions 134
make-up 19
making appointments see
   appointments
Management of Health and Safety
   at Work Regulations
   (1999) 158
manual handling 11–12
Manual Handling Operations Regulations
   (1992) 161
massage techniques 73–4
   effleurage 73
   friction 73
   petrissage 74
   rotary 73
   shaving 154
meche highlights 99
   removing 102
medicated shampoo 71
medulla 77, 81
melanin 97
micro-organisms 56
mint shampoo 71
mirrors 59
moisturising balm 145
moulding/defining crème 88–9
mousse 89
mouth 20

nails 19, 20
neutraliser 107
neutralising 107–8, 111–14
   after the perm 113
   application 112–13
   choosing a neutraliser 111
   faults 113–14
   first rinsing 112
   preparation 112
   rebalancing 111
   second rinsing 113
NVQ 24

obstructions 11
oil shampoo 71

paddle brush 85
pathogens 56
penetrating conditioner 77
perm curlers 55
permanent colour 98
perming 107–14
   how it works 108
   minimise waste 109–10
   protect client/self 108–9
   see also neutralising
perming faults 113
   broken hair 114
   frizzy hair 114
   perm weak and drops 114
   scalp tender/sore/broken 114
   straight hair 114
   straight sections 114
personal
   appearance 19
   behaviour 21
   health and hygiene 20–1
   wellbeing 7, 21
personal development see learning
   and development
personal development plan 24
personal hygiene 69
personal protective equipment (PPE)
   12–13, 109
Personal Protective Equipment (PPE) at
   Work Regulations (1992) 159
petrissage 66, 74, 154
pH balance 66
pH level 107
pheomelanin 98
pigments 97–8
pins 55
plaited/braided extensions 133
plaiting/twisting 117–29
   2-stem twist step-by-step 128–9
   3-stem loose plait 125
   cane rows 126
   cornrowing step-by-step 127
   cornrows 118, 126
   double twists 118
   flat twist step-by-step 128
   French plait 118
   French plait step-by-step 125–6
   hair textures 122
   loose plaits 124–5
   position client/self 118–19
   products 122–3
   sectioning 121
   securing ends of plaits 121
   Senegalese twists 129
   tension 122
   timing of services 120
   tools and equipment 121
plastic capes 13
posture 21, 26
   blow drying 82
   shampoo/conditioning 69
   shaving 147

PPE (personal protective equipment)
   12–13, 109
practice block 117
preventing infection 14–15
Prices Act (1974) 164
products see styling/finishing products
professionalism 24, 27
Provision and Use of Work Equipment
   Regulations (PUWER) (1998) 161

quasi-permanent 98

reception 37–48
   appointment system 37, 45
   appointments 45–8
   asking for help 48
   checklist 39–40
   client care 37, 40–2
   confidentiality 44
   difficult/angry clients 48
   drop in clients 46
   equipment 39
   first impressions 27–8, 38
   greeting clients 42, 46
   handling enquiries 41–2
   keeping clean/tidy 38–9
   keeping stylists informed 42
   recording information 46, 48
   referring enquires 43
   retail products/displays 39
   service timings 47
   stationary 39
   taking messages 43
   telephone 43, 46
referring 43
re-growth colour 99
removing colour 101–4
   emulsifying 102–3
   multiple colours 103–4
   single colour process 103
Reporting of Injuries, Diseases and
   Dangerous Occurrences Regulations
   (RIDDOR) (1995) 18, 161
Resale Prices Act (1964) (1976) 164
respect 25, 29
retail products
   information 39
   keeping clean/tidy 39
   monitoring 39, 40
revenue stream 53, 62
risk 5
   evaluating 6
   reducing 9–16
risk assessment 12
rollers 55
rotary massage 66, 73, 102
round brush 85

safety see health and safety
Sale of Goods Act (1979) and Sale and
   Supply of Goods Act (1994) 163–4

salon
   disposal of waste 58–9
   floors 63
   keeping clean/tidy 53
   layout 9
   mirrors 59
   replenish stock 61–2
   resources 62
   seating 63
   setting up/preparation 54–7
   tidiness 39–40
sectioning
   plaiting/twisting 121
self-assessment 31
semi-permanent colour 98
Senegalese twists 117, 129
serum 88–9, 123
service timings 47
setting rollers 55
sewn-in extensions 133
   removing 143
shampoo
   clarifying 71
   economical use of 70
   how it works 67
   medicated 71
   types of 71
shampooing 66–76
   checklist 70–1
   effleurage 73
   following instructions 72
   friction 73
   massage techniques 73–4
   petrissage 74
   positioning client/self 68–9
   products and equipment 72
   rinsing/finishing 75
   rotary 73
   step by step 74–5
   timing 70
   water flow and temperature 75
sharp items
   disposal of 11, 59
sharps 5
sharps box 5, 11
shaving 145–56
   bowls/mugs 149
   brushes 148–9
   cleaning equipment 149–50
   cleansing and exfoliating skin 153
   gowning/positioning client 146–7
   hot and cold towels 153–4
   lathering 154–6
   massage techniques 154
   posture 147
   problems 156
   sponges 149
   sterilisation 150
   tools and equipment 148–50

shaving brush 148–9
shaving products 152
shoes 19
short hair
   blow drying 92–3
skin
   cleansing and exfoliating 153
slipping hazard 13–14
soya shampoo 71
spillages 14
stationary 39
steamer 60–1, 72
sterilisation 5, 15, 53
   autoclave 15
   chemical 15
   ultraviolet (UV) radiation 15
stock
   monitoring 70
   replenishing 61–2
   rotation 53, 62
structure of hair 77
styling tools 60
styling/finishing products
   clay 89
   fixing spray 123
   gel 89, 123
   glaze 89, 123
   hairspray 88, 90
   moulding/defining crème 88–9
   mousse 89
   serum 88–9, 123
   wax 89–90, 123
surface conditioner 77
surface tension 67
synthetic (artificial) extension
      hair 137–8

taking messages 43
targets 33–4
tea tree oil shampoo 71
teamwork 29–30
telephone 43, 46
tension
   plaiting/twisting 122
tone of voice 42
tools and equipment 54–7
   accelerators 60
   basin/backwash 61
   blow dryers 85–6
   brushes 83–5
   diffuser 85
   extension removal 138
   flat clip 121
   grips 55
   hair trap 61
   hood dryer 60, 72
   mirrors 59
   perm curlers 55

pins 55
reception 39
rollers 55
setting up 54–7
shaving bowls/mugs 149
shaving brushes 148–9
shaving tools 148–50
sponges 149
steamer 60–1, 72
styling tools 60
towels 13, 61
trolleys/trays 55–6
wide-tooth comb 82
towels 13, 61
traction alopecia 117, 124, 139
Trades Descriptions Act (1968)
      (1972) 164
trays 55–6
treatment conditioner 77
tripping hazard 13–14
trolleys 55–6
T-section colour 99
twisting hair see plaiting/twisting

ultraviolet (UV) radiation 15

vented brush 84–5
virgin hair 97
virus 56

waste
   disposal 11, 58–9
   minimising 109–10
wax 89–90, 123
wellbeing 7, 21
working effectively 24–35, 110–11
   appraisal/review 32–4
   asking for feedback 31–2
   keeping stylists informed 42
   self-assessment 31
working environment see workplace
working safely 11–18
workplace
   appeal/grievance procedure 34–5
   being responsible 7–8
   health and safety 5–21
   job description 30–4
   limits of authority 30
   teamwork 29–30
   work routines 7
   working safely 11–18
Workplace (Health, Safety and Welfare)
      Regulations (1992) 158–9

young workers at risk 158